D0398844

*Diagnosis and Treatment of Chronic Depression*

# *Diagnosis and Treatment of Chronic Depression*

Edited by

JAMES H. KOCSIS
DANIEL N. KLEIN

*Foreword by Allen J. Frances*



THE GUILFORD PRESS
New York London

A Division of Guilford Publications, Inc.
72 Spring Street, New York, NY 10012



Printed in the United States of America

This book is printed on acid-free paper.

Last digit is print number: 9 8 7 6 5 4 3 2 1

**Library of Congress Cataloging-in-Publication Data**

Diagnosis and treatment of chronic depression / edited by James H. Kocsis, Daniel N. Klein, foreword by Allen J. Frances.
p. cm.
Includes bibliographical references and index.
ISBN 0-89862-849-0
1. Depression, Mental. I. Kocsis, James H. II. Klein, Daniel N.
[DNLM: 1. Depressive Disorder—diagnosis. 2. Depressive Disorder—therapy. WM 171 D5355 1995]
RC537.D474 1995
616.85'27—dc20
DNLM/DLC
for Library of Congress

95-2539
CIP

*To Randy, Alison, James,*
*Eliza, and Maggie.*– J. H. K.

*To Deborah, Benjamin, and Rebecca.*– D. N. K.

*The editors would like to thank and acknowledge Ms. Carmen Fontanes for her help in preparation of the manuscript.*

# Contributors

**John Barnhill, MD,** Department of Psychiatry, Cornell University Medical College, New York, New York

**Allen J. Frances, MD,** Department of Psychiatry, Duke University Medical Center, Durham, North Carolina

**Richard A. Friedman, MD,** Department of Psychiatry, Cornell University Medical College, New York, New York

**Daniel W. Goodman, MD,** Department of Psychiatry, Cornell University Medical College, New York, New York

**Diane L. Hanks, MA,** Department of Psychiatry and Human Behavior, Brown University, Providence, Rhode Island

**Wilma M. Harrison, MD,** Department of Psychiatry, Columbia University College of Physicians and Surgeons, New York, New York

**Martin B. Keller, MD,** Department of Psychiatry and Human Behavior, Brown University, Providence, Rhode Island

**Daniel N. Klein, PhD,** Department of Psychology, State University of New York at Stony Brook, Stony Brook, New York

**James H. Kocsis, MD,** Department of Psychiatry, Cornell University Medical College, New York, New York

**Maria Kovacs, PhD,** Department of Psychiatry, University of Pittsburgh School of Medicine, and Western Psychiatric Institute and Clinic, Pittsburgh, Pennsylvania

**Andrew C. Leon, PhD,** Department of Psychiatry, Cornell University Medical College, New York, New York

**John C. Markowitz, MD,** Department of Psychiatry, Cornell Medical College, New York, New York

**Barbara J. Mason, PhD,** Department of Psychiatry, University of Miami School of Medicine, Miami, Florida

**Robert O. Morgan, PhD,** Miami Veterans Affairs Medical Center, Miami, Florida

**Michael K. Parides, MS,** Department of Psychiatry, Cornell University Medical College, New York, New York

**Andrew G. Renouf, PhD,** Department of Psychiatry, University of Pittsburgh School of Medicine, and Western Psychiatric Institute and Clinic, Pittsburgh, Pennsylvania

**Jonathan W. Stewart, MD,** Department of Psychiatry, Columbia University College of Physicians and Surgeons, New York, New York

**Seth Thompson, MPhil,** Department of Biostatistics, Columbia University, New York, New York

# Foreword

This book on chronic depression is a wonderful summary of the recent advances in our knowledge on this important topic. It also clarifies how much remains unknown and needs to be studied further. The recent surge of research on chronic depression has documented fairly compellingly that it (1) is a prevalent condition in both clinical and community samples; (2) can be assessed reliably in order to both diagnose and measure change; (3) is associated with an increased risk of having or developing a wide variety of other psychiatric disorders; (4) is characterized by considerable depressive symptomatology and impairment in functioning; (5) may have an onset in childhood and, if untreated, may follow a chronic course; (6) is significantly and substantially more responsive to antidepressant medications than to placebos; (7) has a particularly low placebo response rate, which probably accounts in part for its chronicity; and (8) is a condition in which treatment responders may experience a profound and enduring reduction in their depressive symptomatology and functional impairment.

Even more remains relatively unknown about dysthymia, including the following: (1) how best to define and subtype it, both cross-sectionally and longitudinally; (2) how best to understand its relationship to the many other conditions to which it may be a predisposition, an accompaniment, or a consequence; (3) whether to treat it with medication or psychotherapy or both; and (4) how it relates to personality disorders.

Although there has been a long history in psychiatry of observation and description of chronic depression, the systematic research on this condition has been performed for only about 15 years. A few caveats are certainly in order:

- The construct of dysthymia undoubtedly includes a heterogeneity of different etiologies and presentations.
- Much of what passes for the comorbidity of other disorders with dysthymia is probably better understood as the evolution of a complex syndrome with a shared pathogenesis.
- Our current definitions of major depression and dysthymia reinforce what may be a false categorical distinction, namely, that these are separate depressions; it may be more useful to describe depressions more dimensionally and to consider the lifetime course in classifying them.
- It is unwise to assume that the Axis I versus Axis II distinction means that it will someday be possible to determine the degree to which an individual case of dysthymia is more a mood disorder or more a personality disorder. Early-onset dysthymia can be conceptualized both ways, and the distinction between mood disorder and personality disorder may become meaningless in describing this boundary construct.
- The effective treatments for dysthymic disorder are also likely to be multiple and to include various types of medication and psychotherapy, as well as combinations of these.

In the treatment of chronic depression, as in every other aspect of clinical practice, it is often necessary to make treatment decisions in the absence of clearly established and well-researched guidelines. Here are a few rules of thumb based on my own clinical experience:

1. Combined medication and psychotherapy is necessary for the treatment of chronic depression.
2. Treatments (both medication and psychotherapy) will have to be of relatively long duration, although after remission the frequency of therapeutic visits can be reduced.
3. Because patients have often had many inadequate and ineffective previous treatments, they often begin with low expectations, unless they receive a thorough initial psychoeducation about the condition and its treatment.

4. It is important to choose medications and dosages in a way that minimizes noncompliance due to side effects and takes into account the target symptom profile and comorbid conditions.
5. Psychotherapeutic techniques (e.g., cognitive, interpersonal, behavioral) that were developed originally for acute depressions are effective in modified form in the treatment of chronic depression.
6. A focus on superego pathology and the personality trait of perfectionism is often useful.

The chapters you are about to read are uniformly well written, comprehensive, and balanced. They have been prepared by the leading researchers and clinicians in this field and encompass all that is known about chronic depression. Daniel N. Klein begins the book with a lucid discussion of the many problems encountered in classifying chronic depressions and in assessing and diagnosing the individual patient. Andrew G. Renouf and Maria Kovacs discuss dysthymia in childhood and adolescence; their studies have been crucially important in validating adult retrospective memories of lifetime depression and in highlighting the morbidity associated with the early onset of chronic depression. John C. Markowitz outlines the frequent co-occurrence of dysthymic disorder with other conditions and discusses the pathologenic implications of these relationships. Martin B. Keller and Diane L. Hanks shed light on the course and natural history of dysthymic disorder. Barbara J. Mason and her associates indicate how best to assess symptoms and evaluate change, particularly in response to treatment. Richard A. Friedman discusses the serious social and vocational impairments that are often consequent to dysthymia. Daniel W. Goodman and John Barnhill present what is known about family history of dysthymic disorder. Finally, in chapters of great importance to clinicians, Wilma M. Harrison and Jonathan W. Stewart summarize the pharmacotherapy and John C. Markowitz the psychotherapy of dysthymic disorder. The book closes with an overview and forecast by Daniel N. Klein and my old friend and colleague James H. Kocsis, who has probably been the single most important contributor to our understanding of the classification, diagnosis, and treatment of chronic depression.

I have learned a great deal from this book and feel sure you will also find it extremely helpful in diagnosing and treating this commonly encountered, often difficult, but very rewarding group of patients.

ALLEN J. FRANCES

# Contents

CHAPTER ONE

# Diagnosis and Classification of Dysthymic Disorder

DANIEL N. KLEIN

Dysthymic disorder is a syndrome characterized by a pattern of chronic, low-grade depressive symptoms. This condition has attracted considerable controversy since it was first introduced in DSM-III (American Psychiatric Association, 1980). This chapter briefly discusses the antecedents of the construct, outlines the major issues in the diagnosis and classification of dysthymia, and reviews the evidence bearing on these issues.

## Antecedents

The concept of dysthymia is an admixture of three older clinical constructs: neurotic depression, depressive personality, and chronic depression.

### *Neurotic Depression*

The concept of neurotic depression can be traced to the early part of this century when the classical German descriptive psychopathologists attempted to distinguish between "biological" and "psychogenic" forms of mood disorders. In the United States the concept of neurotic depression was embraced by both the Meyerian and psychoanalytic traditions (Klein, Riso, & Anderson, 1993). Over the years this term has been defined in a variety of ways, including nonpsychotic, mild, lacking melancholic features, chronic, precipitated by psychosocial stressors, lacking a biogenetic etiology, and associated with neurotic personality traits (Klerman, Endicott, Spitzer, & Hirschfeld, 1979). Some of these characteristics have been preserved in the DSM-IV (American Psychiatric Association, 1994) construct of dysthymic disorder (e.g., nonpsychotic, mild, and chronic) while others have not (e.g., precipitated by stress).

## Depressive Personality

The concepts of depressive personality and depressive temperament also date back to the classical descriptive psychopathologists (Kraepelin, 1921; Kretschmer, 1936). These concepts were developed to describe a pattern of depressive-like traits that characterized the premorbid personalities of many manic–depressive patients and their relatives (Phillips, Gunderson, Hirschfeld, & Smith, 1990). The concept of depressive personality was subsequently elaborated by Kurt Schneider (1958), who rejected the Kraepelinian notion of a genetic link between depressive personality and the major mood disorders. Depressive personality has also been widely described in the psychoanalytic literature, where it is often linked with the concept of masochistic (self-defeating) personality (i.e., Kernberg's [1988] depressive–masochistic character disorder).

## Chronic Depression

Although cases of chronic depression have long been described, only recently has there been widespread recognition that a substantial proportion of depressives suffer from chronic conditions. This has been fostered in large part by naturalistic follow-up studies indicating that 15% to 20% of major depressions exhibit a chronic course (Keller, Lavori, Rice, Coryell, & Hirschfeld, 1986; Weissman & Klerman, 1977).

## Relationship to Major Depression

When dysthymic disorder was introduced in DSM-III, one of the most controversial aspects was its inclusion in the mood disorders, rather than the personality disorders, section. Although dysthymia is defined by depressive symptoms, critics argued that its characteristically early onset and chronic, sometimes lifelong, course is more suggestive of a personality disorder than a classical mood disorder (Frances, 1980; Frances & Cooper, 1981; Phillips et al., 1990). In addition, the earlier editions of the American Psychiatric Association's *Diagnostic and Statistical Manual of Mental Disorders* (DSM-I and DSM-II) and the International Classification of Diseases had traditionally classified affective personalities as personality disorders. Hence, a central issue in the literature on the classification of dysthymia has been the validity of conceptualizing dysthymia as a form of mood disorder (Akiskal, 1983; Kocsis & Frances, 1987).

### *Comorbidity with Major Depression*

One of the most consistent sources of support for the relationship of dysthymia to the major mood disorders stems from studies of its co-occurrence with major depression. High rates of comorbidity between dysthymia and major depression have been reported in studies of inpatients, outpatients, and community samples and of children, adolescents, and adults (Asarnow & Ben-Meir, 1988; Ferro, Carlson, Greyson, & Klein, 1994; Keller & Shapiro, 1982; Klein, Taylor, Dickstein, & Harding, 1988b; Kocsis, Markowitz, & Prien, 1990; Kovacs, Feinberg, Crouse-Novak, Paulauskas, & Finkelstein, 1984; Lewinsohn, Rohde, Seeley, & Hops, 1991; Weissman, Leaf, Bruce, & Florio, 1988). A representative study is the recent DSM-IV Mood Disorders Field Trial, which involved administering structured diagnostic interviews to 524 depressives from inpatient, outpatient, and community settings (Keller et al., in press). Of the 190 dysthymics in the sample, 62% met criteria for a current episode of major depression and 80% for lifetime major depression.

This high comorbidity can be attributed to two factors. First, the DSM-III, DSM-III-R (American Psychiatric Association, 1987), and DSM-IV criteria for dysthymia identify a more symptomatically severe condition than is commonly recognized. For example, persons meeting criteria for dysthymia exhibit, on average, 2 to 3 times as many symptoms as are required for the diagnosis (Klein et al., 1993, in press). At the same time, the current criteria for major depression have a low threshold, meaning that a number of milder cases of depression that would not traditionally have been classified as a major mood disorder are now diagnosed as such (Klein, 1990b; Kocsis, 1993). As a result, most patients meeting criteria for dysthymia experience periodic exacerbations in which they also meet criteria for major depression.

## Family, Biological, and Pharmacological Response Studies

As reviewed in greater detail in subsequent chapters, family, biological, and pharmacological treatment studies also support a relationship between dysthymia and major depression. As of yet, there are no published family studies of dysthymia, that is, studies in which the relatives of dysthymics are directly evaluated for a history of psychopathology. However, several studies have reported family history data based on dysthymics' reports about their relatives (see Chapter 7, this volume). These studies indicate that dysthymics exhibit rates of mood disorders in first-degree relatives that are similar to, or even higher than, those of major depressives (Klein, Taylor, et al., 1988b; Rosenthal, Akiskal, Scott-Strauss, Rosenthal, & David, 1981). Several studies have also addressed this issue from the other direction, namely, by examining the rates of dysthymia in the relatives of patients with major depression. Most of these studies have reported higher rates of dysthymia in the relatives of major depressives than in the relatives of controls (Klein, Clark, Dansky, & Margolis, 1988; Weissman et al., 1984).

Biological and treatment studies have provided further support for the relationship between dysthymia and major depression (see Chapter 8, this volume; Howland, 1991; Howland & Thase, 1991; Miller & Yee, 1994). For example, Akiskal et al. (1980) reported that at least a subgroup of dysthymics exhibit shortened rapid-eye-movement (REM) latencies, a robust (although not entirely specific) correlate of major depression. Suggestive evidence has also been reported for the dexamethasone suppression test (DST) and the thyrotropin-releasing hormone (TRH) stimulation test (Rihmer & Szadoczky, 1993).

In addition, several studies have reported that dysthymics exhibit a significantly better response to antidepressants than to placebo (Hellerstein et al., 1993; Kocsis et al., 1988; Stewart et al., 1989). The Hellerstein et al. (1993) study is particularly noteworthy, since it excluded dysthymics who were currently experiencing a superimposed major depressive episode.

While the family history, biological marker, and treatment response data all suggest that there is a close relationship between dysthymia and major depression, it should be noted that this literature still suffers from several gaps and limitations. Perhaps most importantly, most of these studies have failed to distinguish between dysthymics with concurrent major depression and those without it, and none have included a group of dysthymics with no lifetime history of major depression. Hence, the resemblance between dysthymia and major depression could be due to comorbid major depression in the dysthymics. Because only a small proportion of dysthymics have never experienced a major depressive episode, it is extremely difficult to obtain a sufficient number of "pure" dysthymics to address this issue.

## Follow-Up Studies

Further support for the relationship between dysthymia and major depression comes from evidence that dysthymics with no prior history of major depression are at increased risk for developing major depression over time (see Chapter 4, this volume, for a review). While a number of follow-up studies of dysthymics have been reported (Barrett, 1984; Gonzales, Lewinsohn, & Clarke, 1985; Keller, Lavori, Endicott, Coryell, & Klerman, 1983; Kovacs et al., 1984; McCullough et al., 1988; Sievewright & Tyrer, 1990; Wells, Burnham, Rogers, Hays, & Camp, 1992), most have included patients with past or concurrent major depression. There has been one recent exception, however. Using data from the Epidemiologic Catchment Area Study, Horwath, Johnson, Klerman, and Weissman (1992) found that dysthymics with no prior history of major depression were 5.5 times more likely to experience a major depressive episode over the course of a 1-year follow-up than were subjects without a history of dysthymia or major depression, a highly significant increase.

## *Distinct Disorders or Different Phases of a Single Process?*

The evidence for the relationship between dysthymia and major depression raises another, perhaps more difficult, issue. Given this close relationship, and in particular the high comorbidity between dysthymia and major depression, are there two distinct disorders, as is implied by the existence of separate diagnostic categories in DSM-IV and by use of the term *comorbidity*? Or are dysthymia and major depression simply different phases of a single condition that tends to wax and wane over time (Keller & Lavori, 1984; Angst & Wicki, 1990)?

Demonstrating that two syndromes are qualitatively distinct, as opposed to differing on a quantitative dimension such as severity, is an extremely difficult undertaking (Klein & Riso, 1993). Two types of evidence that might support the distinctiveness of dysthymia in at least a preliminary fashion, however, include (1) data demonstrating that dysthymics exhibit a pattern of symptomatology that is qualitatively different from that of major depressives and (2) data indicating specificity of familial transmission.

Simply finding higher rates of occurrence of particular symptoms among major depressives than among dysthymics would not provide very strong support for dysthymia's distinctiveness, since major depression is traditionally regarded as a more severe disorder. Finding that dysthymics exhibit higher rates of specific symptoms, however, would provide some support for this position. A number of studies have compared dysthymics to major depressives on the frequency of specific depressive symptoms (Berrios & Bulbena-Villarasa, 1990; Klein et al., 1993, in press; Kocsis, Voss, Mann, & Frances, 1986; Lindal & Stefansson, 1991; Steer, Beck, Brown, & Berchick, 1987). These studies vary with respect to the number of symptoms that discriminate the two groups. However, none of the studies found a significantly higher rate of occurrence of any depressive symptom among the dysthymics than among major depressives.

A second type of evidence bearing on the distinctiveness of dysthymia is specificity of familial aggregation. To demonstrate such specificity, it would be necessary to demonstrate that (1) dysthymia is more common in the relatives of dysthymics than in the relatives of episodic major depressives and (2) that episodic major depression is more common in the relatives of episodic major depressives than in the relatives of dysthymics. There are no data currently available that adequately address this issue. However, a recent study reported data on the rates of occurrence of episodic and chronic depressive conditions in the adolescent and young adult offspring of inpatients with primary major depression (Klein, Clark, et al., 1988; Klein et al., 1993). This study found a significantly higher rate of chronic depression (primarily dysthymia and major depression superimposed on dysthymia [double depression]) in the offspring of parents with chronic major and double depression than in the offspring of parents with episodic major depression. However, the offspring of chronic depressives also exhibited a slightly higher rate of episodic depressions, suggesting that there is greater familial aggregation of both chronic and episodic forms of depression in the families of chronically depressed patients. Thus, at this point, the limited evidence available from clinical and family studies suggests that there are few qualitative differences between dysthymia and major depression.

## Relationship to Personality Disorders

As indicated earlier, one of the central issues in the classification of dysthymia is whether it is best conceptualized as a form of mood or of personality disorder. The mounting evidence of a strong link between dysthymia and major depression has rendered increasingly untenable the Schneiderian view that characterological depressions are unrelated to the major mood disorders. However, a number of further issues regarding the relationship between dysthymia and the personality disorders remain.

## Should Dysthymia Be Classified on Axis I or Axis II?

Although there is a growing consensus that dysthymia is closely related to the major mood disorders, many investigators continue to believe that dysthymia should be classified as an Axis II disorder on the basis of its characteristically early onset and chronic course. Indeed, a precedent for classifying Axis I spectrum disorders on Axis II exists in schizotypal personality disorder. The critical issue in this debate concerns the definition of personality disorder and the criteria for distinguishing Axis I and II disorders. Personality disorders are typically defined as enduring conditions that are manifested by early adulthood. Given a strict and consistent application of this definition, dysthymia (in at least its early-onset form) indeed appears to belong on Axis II. However, many other disorders whose position on Axis I is rarely questioned also meet this definition (e.g., obsessive–compulsive disorder, social phobia, alcoholism, schizophrenia). Thus, the problem of dysthymia's position in the nosology is unlikely to be resolved until more satisfactory definitions of what constitutes syndromal (Axis I) and personality disorders are developed.

## The Relationship between Dysthymia and Depressive Personality

The DSM construct of dysthymia emphasizes persistent depressive symptoms, often of a vegetative nature. This contrasts with the classical clinical concept of depressive personality, which emphasizes a particular constellation of personality traits, for example, gloominess, pessimism, submissiveness (Phillips et al., 1990). As a result, several investigators have recently argued that these two constructs, although overlapping, are not isomorphic and that the DSM does not provide a category for individuals with a depressive character structure but without the persistent depressive symptoms necessary to qualify for a diagnosis of dysthymia (Akiskal, 1989; Frances & Cooper, 1981; Goldstein & Anthony, 1988; Gunderson, 1983; Kernberg, 1988).

Several recent studies using both clinical and community samples have reported data addressing this issue (Hirschfeld, Holzer, & Shea, 1992; Klein, 1990a; Klein & Miller, 1993; Phillips

& Gunderson, 1992). All of these studies have reported that although there is a significant association between DSM-III-R dysthymia and the depressive personality, the degree of overlap is modest and that the majority of individuals meeting criteria for one of these conditions do not meet criteria for both. Interestingly, individuals with depressive personality but no lifetime history of mood disorder have an elevated rate of occurrence of mood disorder in their first-degree relatives (Klein & Miller, 1993). This indicates that depressive personality may be part of a spectrum of mood disorders that includes dysthymia and major depression (Akiskal, 1989).

## The Relationship between Dysthymia and Existing Axis II Conditions

Finally, dysthymia has also been viewed as a nonspecific consequence of a variety of chronic life stressors and physical and mental disorders, particularly the personality disorders. The aforementioned studies supporting a link between dysthymia and the major mood disorders are inconsistent with this position. However, there is evidence for an association between dysthymia and the personality disorders, suggesting the need for more complex models that include links between dysthymia and both the major mood disorders and personality disorders.

A number of studies have reported data on the prevalence of Axis II disorders in dysthymics (e.g., Akiskal et al., 1980; Alnaes & Torgerson, 1991; Fabrega, Mezzich, Mezzich, & Coffman, 1986; Flick, Roy-Byrne, Cowley, Shores, & Dunner, 1993; Klein, Taylor, et al., 1988b; Kocsis et al., 1986; Koenigsberg, Kaplan, Gilmore, & Cooper, 1985; Marin, Kocsis, Frances, & Klerman, 1993; Markowitz, Moran, Kocsis, & Frances, 1992; Roy, Sutton, & Pickar, 1985; Sanderson, Wetzler, Beck, & Betz, 1992; Tyrer et al., 1990; Zimmerman & Coryell, 1989). These studies have varied considerably with regard to sample definition, population type, nature of comparison groups, and measures of personality disorders. Therefore, it is not surprising that they have produced conflicting findings. Nonetheless, the majority of studies have indicated that dysthymia, in comparison to other Axis I conditions, is associated with an increased rate of occurrence of a number of personality disorders (particularly borderline personality disorder and avoidant personality disorder). Importantly, one of these studies (Zimmerman & Coryell, 1989) employed a nonclinical sample, ruling out referral bias (Berkson's fallacy) as an explanation for the high rate of comorbidity. In addition, another study reported data suggesting that dysthymics may have an increased rate of personality disorders in their relatives (Klein, Taylor, et al., 1988b). This suggests that the increased rate of Axis II comorbidity is not simply a complication of having an early-onset chronic depression. While a number of potential methodological confounds must still be ruled out (e.g., interviewers were not blind to subjects' Axis I diagnoses; chronic depression may lead to overreporting of negative personal attributes; and the criteria for dysthymia and several Axis II conditions overlap), these data suggest that dysthymia may be significantly associated with at least several personality disorders.

There are a number of models that could potentially account for these data (Klein & Riso, 1993). Several of the more plausible, given the existing data, include the following: (1) Dysthymia is heterogeneous, with distinct affective and characterological subgroups (Akiskal, 1983). (2) Chronic depression and personality disorders arise from shared etiological processes (e.g., serotonergic dysregulation or early parental abuse and neglect). (3) Dysthymia and personality disorder are independent conditions that co-occur because the risk factors associated with each of the disorders have an increased prevalence in the same subgroups, or strata, of the population (population stratification); for example, since parental depression is a risk factor for dysthymia in offspring and marital discord may be a risk factor for some personality disorders in children, the common co-occurrence of depression and marital discord in families could lead to increased comorbidity of depression and personality disorders in the offspring of these families.

## Heterogeneity or Subtypes

The DSM-III criteria for dysthymic disorder defined a relatively heterogeneous group of patients. In DSM-III-R a number of distinctions were introduced in an effort to create more homogeneous subgroups. For the most part, these distinctions have been retained in DSM-IV. First, following Akiskal's (1983) typology of chronic depressions, a chronic subtype of major depression was created for individuals whose chronic depressions appear to represent a failure to recover from a major depressive episode rather than a true dysthymia. In DSM-III-R the key distinction between dysthymia and chronic major depression concerns the mode of onset. If the chronic depressive condition began with a full-syndromal major depressive episode, the diagnosis is chronic major depression. However, if the onset was milder and more insidious and it took at least 2 years to reach the proportions of a full major depressive episode, the diagnosis is dysthymia.

While there is some literature on the acute–chronic distinction in major depression, there are virtually no data on the validity of the distinction between chronic major depression and dysthymia. Since this distinction is based almost entirely on patients' reports of the onset of chronic depression, something that generally occurred many years earlier, often in childhood, it is particularly important to determine whether this distinction can be made reliably.

DSM-III-R also introduced two subtyping distinctions within dysthymia: early (before age 21) versus late (age 21 or later) onset and primary versus secondary. The three studies that have compared early- and late-onset dysthymics have yielded inconsistent findings (Klein, Taylor, Dickstein, & Harding, 1988a; McCullough et al., 1990; Shore et al., 1992). In one study the early-onset group had significantly greater comorbidity, a higher rate of mood disorders in their relatives, and higher levels of depressive symptomatology in a 6-month follow-up (Klein, Taylor, et al., 1988a). The other two studies examined a smaller range of variables and found few differences between the groups, although in one of the studies the early-onset subgroup was reported to have a significantly longer duration of illness (Shore et al., 1992).

The primary–secondary dysthymia distinction in DSM-III-R is based on a judgment regarding etiology. If the clinician believes that the dysthymia is caused by a preexisting chronic nonaffective Axis I or Axis III disorder, it is diagnosed as secondary. Otherwise, it is designated as primary. This contrasts with the primary–secondary distinction in the Feighner et al. (1972) and Research Diagnostic Criteria (Spitzer, Endicott, & Robins, 1978) systems, which is based strictly on chronology. Given the possible nonspecificity of chronic low-grade depression, the primary–secondary distinction in DSM-III-R appears to be important. Unfortunately, there are no data available on the reliability of clinicians' judgments of the etiological relationship between dysthymia and other Axis I and Axis III disorders or on the validity of this subtyping distinction. Thus this subtype was dropped from DSM-IV.

Finally, Akiskal (1983) proposed subdividing primary early-onset dysthymia into subaffective and character-spectrum subtypes. In his study a group of early-onset dysthymics were divided on the basis of response to open trials of antidepressants. The responders were characterized by depressive personality traits, a family history of mood disorders, shortened REM latency, and an increased rate of pharmacologically mobilized hypomania. In contrast, the nonresponders were characterized by sociopathic and histrionic personality traits, early object loss, a family history of alcoholism, and normal REM latency. On the basis of these differences, Akiskal (1983) proposed criteria for subaffective dysthymia that emphasized the presence of selected depressive symptoms (e.g., psychomotor retardation, hypersomnia) and depressive personality traits. Several subsequent studies have provided preliminary support for Akiskal's typology (Hauri & Sateia, 1984; Rihmer, 1990; Rimer & Szadoczky, 1993), but negative results have also been reported (Murphy & Checkley, 1990). Unfortunately, all of these studies have significant methodological limitations. Hence, there remains a need for better studies of the subaffective–character spectrum distinction.

## Summary and Conclusions

To summarize, the DSM-IV construct of dysthymia is the product of several overlapping clinical concepts and traditions. While the decision to classify dysthymia as a mood, rather than a personality, disorder was controversial, a growing body of evidence indicates that there is a strong link between dysthymia and major depression. Indeed, at this point there is little evidence suggesting that dysthymia and major depression exhibit any significant qualitative differences. Instead, they may represent different phases of the same process.

Dysthymia also appears to be significantly associated with

several Axis II disorders, particularly borderline personality disorder and avoidant personality disorder. However, the cause of these associations is currently unclear.

Although dysthymia and the classical concept of the depressive personality overlap, the two constructs do not appear to be equivalent. Thus, there appears to be a group of individuals with prominent depressive personality traits who lack the persistent symptoms needed to qualify for a diagnosis of dysthymia. Interestingly, these individuals appear to have a familial relationship to the major mood disorders.

Finally, several subtyping distinctions have been introduced to reduce the heterogeneity of dysthymia. Unfortunately, sufficient data on their reliability and validity are not available to permit an adequate evaluation.

## Acknowledgment

Preparation of this chapter was supported in part by NIMH Grant No. RO1 MH45757. This chapter is based in part on Klein and Kelly (1993). Copyright 1993 by Slack, Inc. Adapted by permission.

## References

Akiskal, H. S. (1983). Dysthymic disorder: Psychopathology of proposed chronic depressive subtypes. *American Journal of Psychiatry, 140,* 11–20.

Akiskal, H. S. (1989). Validating affective personality types. In L. N. Robins & J. E. Barrett (Eds.), *The validity of psychiatric diagnosis* (pp. 217–227). New York: Raven Press.

Akiskal, H. S., Rosenthal, T. L., Haykal, R. F., Lemmi, H., Rosenthal, R. H., & Scott-Strauss, A. (1980). Characterological depressions: Clinical and sleep EEG findings separating "subaffective dysthymias" from "character spectrum disorders." *Archives of General Psychiatry, 37,* 777–783.

Alnaes, R., & Torgerson, S. (1991). Personality and personality disorders among patients with various affective disorders. *Journal of Personality Disorders, 5,* 107–121.

American Psychiatric Association. (1980). *Diagnostic and statistical manual of mental disorders* (3rd ed.). Washington, DC: Author.

American Psychiatric Association. (1987). *Diagnostic and statistical manual of mental disorders* (3rd ed., rev.). Washington, DC: Author.

American Psychiatric Association. (1994). *Diagnostic and statistical manual of mental disorders* (4th ed.). Washington, DC: Author.

Angst, J., & Wicki, W. (1990). The Zurich Study: XI. Is dysthymia a separate form of depression? Results of the Zurich Cohort Study. *European Archives of Psychiatry and Clinical Neuroscience, 240*, 349–354.

Asarnow, J., & Ben-Meir, S. (1988). Children with schizophrenia spectrum and depressive disorders: A comparative study of premorbid adjustment, onset pattern, and severity of impairment. *Journal of Child Psychology and Psychiatry, 29*, 477–488.

Barrett, J. E. (1984). Naturalistic change after 2 years in neurotic depressive disorders (RDC categories). *Comprehensive Psychiatry, 25*, 404–418.

Berrios, G. E., & Bulbena-Villarasa, A. (1990). The Hamilton Depression Scale and the numerical description of the symptoms of depression. In P. Bech & A. Coppen (Eds.), *The Hamilton scales* (pp. 80–92). Berlin: Springer-Verlag.

Fabrega, H., Mezzich, J. E., Mezzich, A. C., & Coffman, G. A. (1986). Descriptive validity of DSM-III depressions. *Journal of Nervous and Mental Disease, 174*, 573–584.

Feighner, J. P., Robins, E., Guze, S. B., Woodruff, R. A., Winokur, G., & Munoz, R. (1972). Diagnostic criteria for use in psychiatric research. *Archives of General Psychiatry, 26*, 57–63.

Ferro, T., Carlson, G. A., Grayson, P., & Klein, D. N. (1994). Depressive disorders: Distinctions in children. *Journal of the American Academy of Child and Adolescent Psychiatry, 33*, 664–670.

Flick, S. N., Roy-Byrne, P. P., Cowley, D. S., Shores, M. M., & Dunner, D. L. (1993). DSM-III-R personality disorders in a mood and anxiety disorders clinic: Prevalence, comorbidity, and correlates. *Journal of Affective Disorders, 27*, 71–79.

Frances, A. (1980). The DSM-III personality disorders section: A commentary. *American Journal of Psychiatry, 137*, 1050–1054.

Frances, A., & Cooper, A. M. (1981). Descriptive and dynamic psychiatry: A perspective on DSM-III. *American Journal of Psychiatry, 138*, 1198–1202.

Goldstein, W. N., & Anthony, R. N. (1988). The diagnosis of depression and the DSMs. *American Journal of Psychotherapy, 42*, 180–196.

Gonzales, L. R., Lewinsohn, P. M., & Clarke, G. N. (1985). Longitudinal follow-up of unipolar depressives: An investigation of predictors of relapse. *Journal of Consulting and Clinical Psychology, 53*, 461–469.

Gunderson, J. (1983). DSM-III diagnoses of personality disorders. In J. P.

Frosch (Ed.), *Current perspectives on personality disorders* (pp. 20–39). Washington, DC: American Psychiatric Press.

Hauri, P., & Sateia, M. J. (1984). REM sleep in dysthymic disorders. *Sleep Research, 13,* 119.

Hellerstein, D. J., Yanowitch, P., Rosenthal, J., Samstag, L. W., Maurer, M., Kasch, K., Burrows, L., Poster, M., Cantillon, M., & Winston, A. (1993). A randomized double-blind study of fluoxetine versus placebo in the treatment of dysthymia. *American Journal of Psychiatry, 150,* 1169–1175.

Hirschfeld, R. M. A., Holzer, C. P. III, & Shea, M. T. (1992, May). *Depressive personality: Results of the DSM-IV Mood Disorders Field Trial.* Paper presented at the annual meeting of the American Psychiatric Association, Washington, DC.

Horwath, E., Johnson, J., Klerman, G. L., & Weissman, M. M. (1992). Depressive symptoms as relative and attributable risk factors for first-onset major depression. *Archives of General Psychiatry, 49,* 817–823.

Howland, R. H. (1991). Pharmacotherapy of dysthymia. *Journal of Clinical Psychopharmacology, 11,* 83–92.

Howland, R. H., & Thase, M. E. (1991). Biological studies of dysthymia. *Biological Psychiatry, 30,* 283–304.

Keller, M. B., Klein, D. N., Hirschfeld, R. M. A., Koscis, J. H., McCullough, J. P., Miller, I., First, M. B., Holzer, C. P. III, Keitner, G. I., Marin, D. B., & Shea, M. T. (in press). DSM-IV Mood Disorders Field Trial investigation results. *American Journal of Psychiatry.*

Keller, M. B., & Lavori, P. W. (1984). Double depression, major depression, and dysthymia: Distinct entities or different phases of a single disorder. *Psychopharmacology Bulletin, 20,* 399–402.

Keller, M. B., Lavori, P. W., Endicott, J., Coryell, W., & Klerman, G. L. (1983). "Double depression": Two-year follow-up. *American Journal of Psychiatry, 140,* 689–694.

Keller, M. B., Lavori, P. W., Rice, J., Coryell, W., & Hirschfeld, R. M. A. (1986). The persistent risk of chronicity in recurrent episodes of nonbipolar major depression: A prospective follow-up. *American Journal of Psychiatry, 143,* 24–28.

Keller, M. B., & Shapiro, R. W. (1982). Double depression: Superimposition of acute depressive episodes on chronic depressive disorders. *American Journal of Psychiatry, 139,* 438–442.

Kernberg, O. F. (1988). Clinical dimensions of masochism. *Journal of the American Psychoanalytic Association, 36,* 1005–1029.

Klein, D. N.(1990a). Depressive personality: Reliability, validity, and relation to dysthymia. *Journal of Abnormal Psychology, 99,* 412–421.

Klein, D. N. (1990b). Symptom criteria and family history in major depression. *American Journal of Psychiatry, 147,* 850- 854.

Klein, D. N., Clark, D. C., Dansky, L., & Margolis, E. (1988). Dysthymia in the offspring of parents with primary unipolar affective disorder. *Journal of Abnormal Psychology, 97,* 265–274.

Klein, D. N., & Kelly, H. S. (1993). Diagnosis and classification of dysthymia. *Psychiatric Annals, 23,* 609–616.

Klein, D. N., Kocsis, J. H., McCullough, J. P., Holzer, C. P. III, Keller, M. B., Hirschfeld, R. M. A., First, M. B., Miller, I., Keitner, G. I., Marin, D. B., & Shea, M. T. (in press). Symptomatology in dysthymia and major depression. *Psychiatric Clinics of North America.*

Klein, D. N., & Miller, G. A. (1993). Depressive personality in nonclinical subjects. *American Journal of Psychiatry, 150,* 1718–1724.

Klein, D. N., & Riso, L. P. (1993). Psychiatric disorders: Problems of boundaries and comorbidity. In C. G. Costello (Ed.), *Basic issues in psychopathology* (pp. 19–66). New York: Guilford Press.

Klein, D. N., Riso, L. P., & Anderson, R. L. (1993). DSM-III-R dysthymia: Antecedents and underlying assumptions. In L. J. Chapman, J. P. Chapman, & D. C. Fowles (Eds.), *Progress in experimental personality and psychopathology research* (Vol. 16, pp. 222–253). New York: Springer.

Klein, D. N., Taylor, E. T., Dickstein, S., & Harding, K. (1988a). The early–late onset distinction in DSM-III-R dysthymia. *Journal of Affective Disorders, 14,* 25–33.

Klein, D. N., Taylor, E. T., Dickstein, S., & Harding, D. (1988b). Primary early-onset dysthymia: Comparison with primary nonbipolar nonchronic major depression on demographic, clinical, familial, personality, and socioenvironmental characteristics and short-term outcome. *Journal of Abnormal Psychology, 97,* 387–398.

Klerman, G. L., Endicott, J., Spitzer, R. L., & Hirschfeld, R. M. A. (1979). Neurotic depressions: A systematic analysis of multiple criteria and meanings. *American Journal of Psychiatry, 136,* 57–61.

Kocsis, J. H. (1993). DSM-IV "Major Depression": Are more stringent criteria needed? *Depression, 1* 24–28.

Kocsis, J. H., & Frances, A. J. (1987). A critical discussion of DSM-III dysthymic disorder. *American Journal of Psychiatry, 144,* 1534–1542.

Kocsis, J. H., Frances, A. J., Voss, C., Mann, J. J., Mason, B. J., & Sweeney, J. (1988). Imipramine treatment for chronic depression. *Archives of General Psychiatry, 45,* 253–257.

Kocsis, J. H., Markowitz, J. C., & Prien, R. F. (1990). Comorbidity of dysthymic disorder. In J. D. Maser & C. R. Cloninger (Eds.), *Comorbidity in anxiety and mood disorders* (pp. 317–328). Washington, DC: American Psychiatric Press.

Kocsis, J. H., Voss, C., Mann, J. J., & Frances, A. (1986). Chronic depression: Demographic and clinical characteristics. *Psychopharmacology Bulletin, 22,* 192–195.

Koenigsberg, H. W., Kaplan, R. D., Gilmore, M. M., & Cooper, A. M. (1985). The relationship between syndrome and personality disorder in DSM-III-R: Experience with 2,462 patients. *American Journal of Psychiatry, 142,* 207–212.

Kovacs, M., Feinberg, T. L., Crouse-Novak, M. A., Paulauskas, S. L., & Finkelstein, R. (1984). Depressive disorders in childhood: I. A longitudinal prospective study of characteristics and recovery. *Archives of General Psychiatry, 41,* 229–237.

Kraepelin, E. (1921). *Manic depressive insanity and paranoia.* Edinburgh: E. & S. Livingstone.

Kretschmer, E. (1936). *Physique and character* (2nd ed.). London: Routledge.

Lewinsohn, P. M., Rohde, P., Seeley, J. R., & Hops, H. (1991). Comorbidity of unipolar depression: I. Major depression with dysthymia. *Journal of Abnormal Psychology, 100,* 205–213.

Lindal, E., & Stefansson, J. G. (1991). The frequency of depressive symptoms in a general population with reference to DSM-III. *International Journal of Social Psychiatry, 37,* 233–241.

Marin, D. B., Kocsis, J. H., Frances, A. J., & Klerman, G. L. (1993). Personality disorders in dysthymia. *Journal of Personality Disorders, 7,* 223–231.

Markowitz, J. C., Moran, M. M., Kocsis, J. H., & Frances, A. J. (1992). Prevalence and comorbidity of dysthymic disorder among psychiatric outpatients. *Journal of Affective Disorders, 24,* 63–71.

McCullough, J. P., Braith, J. A., Chapman, R. C., Kasnetz, M. D., Carr, K. F., Cones, J. H., Fielo, J., & Roberts, W. C. (1990). Comparison of dysthymia major and non-major depressives. *Journal of Nervous and Mental Disease, 178,* 611–612.

McCullough, J. P., Kasnetz, M. D., Braith, J. A., Carr, K. F., Cones, J. H., Fielo, J., & Martelli, J. F. (1988). A longitudinal study of an untreated sample of predominantly late-onset characterological dysthymia. *Journal of Nervous and Mental Disease, 176,* 658–667.

Miller, G. A., & Yee, C. M. (1994). Risk for severe psychopathology: Psychometric screening and psychophysiological assessment. In J. R. Jennings, P. K. Ackles, & M. G. H. Coles (Eds.), *Advances in psychophysiology* (Vol. 5, pp. 1–54). London: Jessica Kingsley.

Murphy, D., & Checkley, S. A. (1990). Dysthymia presenting to the emergency clinic of the Maudsley Hospital. In S. W. Burton & H. S. Akiskal (Eds.), *Dysthymic disorder* (pp. 37–48). London: Gaskell.

Phillips, K. A., & Gunderson, J. G. (1992, May). *An empirical study of the depressive personality*. Paper presented at the annual meeting of the American Psychiatric Association, Washington, DC.

Phillips, K. A., Gunderson, J. G., Hirschfeld, R. M. A., & Smith, L. E. (1990). A review of the depressive personality. *American Journal of Psychiatry*, *147*, 830–837.

Rihmer, Z. (1990). Dysthymia: A clinician's perspective. In S. W. Burton & H. S. Akiskal (Eds.), *Dysthymic disorder* (pp. 112–124). London: Gaskell.

Rihmer, Z., & Szadoczky, E. (1993). Dexamethasone suppression test and TRH-TSH test in subaffective dysthymia and character-spectrum disorder. *Journal of Affective Disorders*, *28*, 287–291.

Rosenthal, T. L., Akiskal, H. S., Scott-Strauss, A., Rosenthal, R. H., & David, M. (1981). Familial and developmental factors in characterological depressions. *Journal of Affective Disorders*, *3*, 183–192.

Roy, A., Sutton, M., & Pickar, D. (1985). Neuroendocrine and personality variables in dysthymic disorder. *American Journal of Psychiatry*, *142*, 94–97.

Sanderson, W. C., Wetzler, S., Beck, A. T., & Betz, F. (1992). Prevalence of personality disorders in patients with major depression and dysthymia. *Psychiatry Research*, *42*, 93–99.

Schneider, K. (1958). *Psychopathic personalities*. London: Cassell.

Shore, M. M., Glubin, T., Cowley, D. S., Dager, S. R., Roy-Byrne, P. P., & Dunner, D. L. (1992). The relationship between anxiety and depression: A clinical comparison of generalized anxiety disorder, dysthymic disorder, panic disorder, and major depressive disorder. *Comprehensive Psychiatry*, *33*, 237–244.

Sievewright, N., & Tyrer, P. (1990). Relationship of dysthymia to anxiety and other neurotic disorders. In S. W. Burton & H. S. Akiskal (Eds.), *Dysthymic disorder* (pp. 24–36). London: Gaskell.

Spitzer, R. L., Endicott, J., & Robins, E. (1978). *Research Diagnostic Criteria (RDC) for a selected group of functional disorders* (3rd ed.). New York: Biometrics Research, New York State Psychiatric Institute.

Steer, R. A., Beck, A. T., Brown, G., & Berchick, R. J. (1987). Self-reported depressive symptoms that differentiate recurrent-episode major depression from dysthymic disorders. *Journal of Clinical Psychology*, *43*, 246–250.

Stewart, J. W., McGrath, P. J., Quitkin, F. M., Harrison, W., Markowitz, J., Wager, S., & Liebowitz, M. R. (1989). Relevance of DSM-III depressive subtypes and chronicity of antidepressant efficacy in atypical depression: Differential response to phenelzine, imipramine, and placebo. *Archives of General Psychiatry*, *46*, 1080–1087.

Tyrer, P., Sievewright, N., Ferguson, B., Murphy, S., Darling, C., Brothwell, J., Kingdon, D., & Johnson, A. L. (1990). The Nottingham Study of Neurotic Disorder: Relationship between personality status and symptoms. *Psychological Medicine, 20,* 423–431.

Weissman, M. M., Gershon, E. S., Kidd, K. K., Prusoff, B. A., Leckman, J. F., Dibble, E., Hamovit, J., Thompson, W. D., Pauls, D.L., & Guroff, J.J. (1984). Psychiatric disorders in the relatives of probands with affective disorder. *Archives of General Psychiatry, 41,* 13–21.

Weissman, M. M., & Klerman, G. L. (1977). The chronic depressive in the community: Unrecognized and poorly treated. *Comprehensive Psychiatry, 18,* 523–532.

Weissman, M. M., Leaf, P. J., Bruce, M. L., & Florio, L. (1988). Epidemiology of dysthymia in five communities: Rates, risks, comorbidity, and treatment. *American Journal of Psychiatry, 145,* 815–819.

Wells, K. B., Burnham, M. A., Rogers, W., Hays, M., & Camp, P. (1992). The course of depression in adult outpatients: Results from the Medical Outcomes Study. *Archives of General Psychiatry, 49,* 788–794.

Zimmerman, M., & Coryell, W. (1989). DSM-III personality diagnoses in a nonpatient sample: Demographic correlates and comorbidity. *Archives of General Psychiatry, 46,* 682–689.

CHAPTER TWO

# Dysthymic Disorder during Childhood and Adolescence

ANDREW G. RENOUF
MARIA KOVACS

In this chapter we first place the current state of research on dysthymic disorder, or dysthymia, in juveniles within a historical context. Then we summarize the empirical literature regarding its clinical characteristics and prevalence. In the final section of the chapter we make suggestions for future research and discuss several implications for treatment.

As a diagnostic entity, dysthymic disorder is relatively new, originating with DSM-III in 1980 (American Psychiatric Association, 1980). The history of this diagnosis is reviewed in Chapter 1; here we will mention only those issues that are pertinent to the current state of research on youths. Although the label "dysthymic disorder" is recent, this entity has been described and studied under a variety of terms in the past, including minor depression, intermittent depression, and neurotic depression. Indeed, there exists a substantial body of theory and research on this condition. However, the extant information is almost exclusively in relation to adults; our group was one of the first to study dysthymia in children, including its clinical presentation and prognosis (Kovacs, Feinberg, Crouse-Novak, Paulauskas, & Finkelstein, 1984; Kovacs, Feinberg, Crouse-Novak, Paulauskas, Pollock, & Finkelstein, 1984).

The sparsity of research on dysthymia in juveniles may partly reflect the ambiguous nosological pedigree of this diagnostic category. In particular, there has been a long-standing controversy as to whether dysthymia is a true affective disorder within the same class as unipolar and bipolar depression or if it is a personality disorder (e.g., Chapter 1, this volume; Akiskal, 1991; Kocsis & Frances, 1987). A chronic course during childhood or adolescence has often been thought of as a hallmark of depressive personality (Akiskal, 1983; Winokur, 1979). Possibly, therefore, youths with protracted depressive symptoms may not have been viewed as a population of interest by researchers wishing to study affective disorders. In addition, until the late 1970s, the existence of depressive disorders in childhood was controversial (e.g., Bibring, 1953; Toolan, 1963; Wolfenstein, 1966). Consequently, investigators interested in juvenile depression, who were originally inspired by the strength and consistency of work on depression in adults (Puig-Antich, 1980), probably bypassed the doubly controversial area of early dysthymia.

The debate over the existence of depression in children is over (e.g., Kovacs, Feinberg, Crouse-Novak, Paulauskas, & Finkelstein, 1984; Rutter, Izard, & Read, 1986). Regarding the appropriate classification of dysthymia, Akiskal (1983, 1991) has suggested at least two subtypes: (1) a true affective disorder that is thought to be prodromal to later episodes of uni- and bipolar depressive episodes and (2) a "character-spectrum disorder." Akiskal's formulation has received increasing empirical support from research with adults (e.g., Keller, Lavori, Endicott, Coryell, & Klerman, 1983; Klein, Taylor, Harding, & Dickstein, 1990; Kocsis, Voss, Mann, & Frances, 1986). Indeed, findings with children by our own research group (Kovacs, Akiskal, Gatsonis, & Parrone, 1994; Kovacs, Feinberg, Crouse-Novak, Paulauskas, Pollock, & Finkelstein, 1984), to be discussed later in this chapter, indicate that dysthymia follows a chronic course that is typical of affective disorders. If uncertainty about the diagnostic status of dysthymia has deterred investigators from examining the disorder in children, the accumulating evidence now warrants increased attention to the condition in juveniles. Our findings and those from research with adults support the contention that at least some forms of dysthymia in children are related to major depression and should be classed as an affective rather than a personality disorder.

## Characteristics of Dysthymic Disorder

The information on childhood-onset dysthymia is scant, particularly compared to what we know about early-onset major depression. And yet, the findings have been remarkably consistent across studies that have differed in sampling strategies, methods of data gathering, and diagnostic procedures. Dysthymia in school-age children and in adolescents is distinguished by a comparatively early onset, a protracted duration, a high rate of within-episode as well as subsequent comorbidity, and a long-term course characterized by repeated episodes of affective illness. Furthermore, a familial vulnerability to affective disorders has been associated with very early onset dysthymia. Recent findings also suggest that the disorder is characterized predominantly by psychologic, as opposed to neurovegetative, symptoms.

Much of the information presented in this section derives from our own Pittsburgh Longitudinal Study, the design of which has been described in detail elsewhere (Kovacs, Feinberg, Crouse-Novak, Paulauskas, & Finkelstein, 1984; Kovacs, Feinberg, Crouse-Novak, Paulauskas, Pollock, & Finkelstein, 1984). Subjects were recruited from among referrals to outpatient psychiatric and medical clinics during a 9-year period spanning the late 1970s to late 1980s. In our cohort of children with a psychiatric diagnosis, 23 had a study entry diagnosis of dysthymic disorder, 32 had major depression superimposed on dysthymia, and 60 had major depression. The group of 55 children with the index diagnosis of dysthymia represented an entirely first-episode cohort and included 27 boys and 28 girls, with African-Americans and families of low socioeconomic status being overrepresented relative to the general population.

Psychiatric diagnoses were derived at each assessment from the semistructured, symptom-oriented Interview Schedule for Children (Kovacs, 1985) and its addenda. Both parents and children were interviewed, and only symptoms that reached or exceeded operationally defined levels of severity counted toward a diagnosis. Final diagnoses were consensually assigned by the research clinicians according to DSM-III criteria. There were two common presentations for a diagnosis of *concurrent* dysthymic and major depressive disorder: Either the dysthymic child developed new symptoms that met criteria for major depression (e.g., in addition to the existing dysthymic symptoms, the child developed appetite and sleep disturbance), or the child's dysthymic symptoms changed in severity, and/or previous subclinical symptoms became exacerbated, so as to reach criterion levels for major depression (e.g., an inability to respond with pleasure to praise evolved into pervasive anhedonia). Thus, in the case of "double depression," some symptoms were counted toward both diagnoses. However, even when the chronic mood disturbance appeared to be prodromal to the major depression, it was diagnosed as dysthymic disorder if it met DSM-III criteria. Alternately, a partially remitted major depression, even when chronic, was never diagnosed as dysthymia.

## *Early Onset and Protracted Duration*

Specific information about the age at which dysthymia first develops, as well as in comparison to the age at onset of major depression, suggests that this disorder can declare itself at a relatively early age. Among clinic-based dysthymic children in the Pittsburgh study, the earliest age at onset was 5 years and the mean age at onset was 8.7 years. In comparison, the children whose first affective disorder was major depression were significantly older at its onset, with a mean age of 10.9 years (Kovacs et al., 1994). Similarly, in a community-based sample of adolescents (Lewinsohn, Rohde, Seeley, & Hops, 1991), dysthymia was found to have an onset that was approximately 3 years earlier than the onset of major depression (11 years versus 14 years). Moreover, in depressed youths who were selected according to criteria not directly related to their psychopathology (Keller et al., 1988), as well as in those identified in the aforementioned community sample (Lewinsohn et al., 1991), dysthymia preceded major depression in practically all cases.

One of the unexpected findings about childhood-onset dysthymic disorder was its protracted duration both in clinic-based and non-clinic-based samples, with average episode lengths from about 2.5 years to 5 years. For example, the median time from onset to recovery of dysthymia in the Pittsburgh sample was 4 years (Kovacs et al., 1994) and in a small non-clinic-based sample of youths the median duration was 5 years (Keller et al., 1988). Among 14- to 18-year-old dysthymic adolescents in the community, average episode length at the time of assessment ranged from 2.5 years for youths with pure dysthymia to 3.4 years for those with double depression (Lewinsohn et al., 1991).

In light of the fact that the better-known disorders of childhood, including attention-deficit and conduct disorders, tend to be chronic, a dysthymia lasting 4 years may not appear to be that protracted. However, if a 9-year-old boy develops a dysthymic disorder from which he recovers 4 years later, he will have spent more than 30% of his entire life and over 50% of his school-age years being depressed. Because depression is associated with academic, cognitive, family, and peer problems (Kovacs & Goldston, 1991; Puig-Antich et al., 1985), the protracted lengths of dysthymia are likely to have important negative consequences on young patients' development.

## Comorbidity

The distinction between primary and secondary depression (Spitzer, Endicott, & Robins, 1978) has been important in the study of psychiatric disorders in adults, with most of the interest being on primary depression, that is, depression not preceded by another psychiatric or medical condition. The importance of this distinction in childhood has not been established. Indeed, the fact that a diagnosis of primary as opposed to secondary dysthymia is more likely in children may partly be a function of the nature and age range of the target population and the age at onset of the dysthymia. For example, given the relative youth of the Pittsburgh sample at the time of ascertainment (8 to 13 years old) and the early age of dysthymia onset, it is not surprising that 53% had primary dysthymia (Kovacs et al., 1994). Among older youths with later-onset depression, primary dysthymia may be less prevalent because the risk period for most of the other childhood-onset disorders was prior to onset of the dysthymia.

More recently, the primary–secondary disorder distinction has been subsumed under the rubric of comorbidity, or the co-occurrence of multiple disorders. According to all indicators, dysthymia in childhood is often complicated by comorbid nonaffective as well as major depressive disorders. However, as is consistent with the data on adults, a superimposed major depression is the most prevalent comorbid diagnosis during childhood. Rates of major depression comorbid with dysthymia vary, depending on whether the youths are ascertained because they have major depression or dysthymia and on the point in the natural course of the disorder at which assessment takes place. When cases are ascertained because they have major depression, approximately 30% are found to have an underlying dysthymia. This rate appears to be fairly stable in clinical and nonclinical samples. For example, 35% of the 8- to 13-year-olds with major depression in the Pittsburgh study had an underlying dysthymia; in the Seattle sample of inpatient and outpatient depressed youths, 33% had a preexisting dysthymia (Myers, McCauley, Calderon, & Treder, 1991); and in studies of the offspring of adult patients and normal adult controls, between 24% and 29% of the children with major depression had an underlying dysthymia (Keller et al., 1988; Warner, Weissman, Fendrich, Wickramaratne, & Moreau, 1992, respectively).

When case ascertainment is by the presence of dysthymia, comorbid major depression is evident at a higher rate. In the Pittsburgh study, 58% of the children with dysthymia at study entry had a superimposed major depression. During the subsequent course of the dysthymia, altogether 69% had at least one episode of superimposed major depression (Kovacs et al., 1994). Similarly, in a community sample of 12- to 14-year-old youths with dysthymia, 58% also had major depression (Garrison, Addy, Jackson, McKeown, & Waller, 1992), and in a sample of 14- to 18-year-old dysthymics in the community, 42% already had a major depression at the time of ascertainment (Lewinsohn et al., 1991).

As mentioned, the rates of comorbid nonaffective disorders are also high. In the Pittsburgh sample, 47% of the dysthymic children had comorbid nonaffective disorders that predated the dysthymia and still were present at the time of assessment, most frequently attention-deficit and anxiety disorders (Kovacs et al., 1994). In an inpatient sample of 7- to 13-year-olds with major depression and/or dysthymia, 54% had comorbid nonaffective disorders, with similar rates of comorbidity for the two depressive disorders (Asarnow et al., 1988). Among somewhat older, nonreferred youths with major or double depression, 53% were found to have a preexisting nonaffective disorder (Keller et al., 1988). Likewise, in a community study of older adolescents, those with "pure" dysthymia evidenced a 38% rate of nondepressive lifetime comorbid disorders (Lewinsohn et al., 1991), and dysthymic youths in another epidemiologic study had a 75% rate of comorbidity (Garrison et al., 1992).

What implications does the high rate of comorbid disorders in juveniles with dysthymia have? From a research perspective, comorbidity complicates the characterization of very early-onset dysthymia (Caron & Rutter, 1991). The presence of additional disorders brings into question whether characteristics of dysthymia such as protracted length of episode and poor prognosis are a function of the dysthymia, the comorbid conditions, or an interaction of the two. From a clinical perspective, however, comorbidity appears to be a fact of life. Whether multiple conditions are due to genetic or environmental liability or to an increased sensitivity to psychiatric problems after the initial episode of dysthymia, common sense dictates that there is at least an additive effect in terms of negative psychosocial repercussions. Furthermore, both diagnosis and treatment may be complicated by the presence of comorbid conditions. Alternatively, early diagnosis of dysthymia may also serve to identify individuals at risk for later affective disorders and successful treatment of the dysthymia may have preventive or ameliorative effects on comorbid disorders. In any case, comorbidity must be taken into account when considering the course and treatment of dysthymia in juveniles.

## Long-Term Outcome

Overall, the indications are that children and adolescents with dysthymia have a mixed long-term prognosis. On the one hand, almost all of them eventually recover from the dysthymia; on the other hand, they are at extremely high risk to develop later psychiatric disorders. Overwhelmingly, these disorders are some form of depression or anxiety.

In the Pittsburgh cohort of dysthymic children we found a cumulative probability of .81 over 8.5 years for developing a first-episode major depression subsequent to dysthymic disorder onset. The second and third years of the dysthymia appear to be a period of particularly high risk for the first episode of major depression. In the majority of cases, major depression was superimposed on the dysthymia (in only a few cases did the major depression develop after the index dysthymia remitted). A second episode of major depression has already been observed in a significant proportion of our cohort. Our dysthymic cohort also was at risk for developing bipolar disorders, with a cumulative probability of .21 over 8.5 years (Kovacs et al., 1994). This risk for bipolarity parallels other findings indicating that a subsample of dysthymic adults go on to develop bipolar disorders, sometimes in response to tricyclic antidepressant medication (Akiskal, 1983; Rihmer, Szadoczky, & Arato, 1983).

Only 9% of dysthymic youngsters in the Pittsburgh cohort have not yet developed another psychiatric disorder during an average follow-up interval of 6 years. The data in Table 2.1 provide a summary of the chronologic sequence of new disorders the remaining 91% of dysthymic children developed subsequent to dysthymia onset. This summary of longitudinal course includes only the first five new disorders (because few youths developed more than five different conditions); multiple episodes of the same disorder were not tallied. In addition to revealing high rates of comorbidity, these data also highlight the poor long-term prognosis of very early-onset dysthymia.

Further evidence of a poor prognosis comes from data indicat-

**TABLE 2.1. Chronologic Sequence of DSM-III Psychiatric Disorders after Onset of Dysthymic Disorder**

| | Disorder occurrence | | | | |
|---|---|---|---|---|---|
| DSM-III disorder | First | Second | Third | Fourth | Fifth |
| Major depressive disorder | 42% | 26% | 7% | 2% | – |
| Bipolar disorder | – | 6% | 4% | 2% | 2% |
| Cyclothymic disorder | – | – | 2% | – | – |
| Separation anxiety disorder | 16% | 11% | – | – | – |
| Overanxious disorder | 9% | 2% | 4% | – | – |
| Other anxiety disorder | 2% | 5% | 4% | 2% | 2% |
| Conduct disorder | 16% | 11% | 2% | 2% | – |
| Substance use/abuse disorder | – | 2% | 2% | 4% | – |
| Developmental/personality disorder | 2% | 8% | 6% | – | – |
| Personality disorder | – | 4% | 4% | – | – |
| Attention-deficit disorder | 2% | – | – | – | – |
| Dysthymic disorder, second episode | – | 4% | 4% | 2% | – |
| Other disorder | 2% | – | 2% | 2% | – |
| No disorder | 9% | 27% | 66% | 86% | 96% |

*Note.* Sequence of occurrence of disorders, excluding adjustment disorders, DSM "V" codes, and enuresis or encopresis, from onset of dysthymic disorder to criterion interview by September 1, 1990 ($n$ = 55).

ing that 40% of inpatient children with dysthymia are rehospitalized within the first year of discharge (Asarnow et al., 1988). Children in this inpatient sample who had major depression superimposed on dysthymia appeared to run a higher risk of rehospitalization within the first 2 years after initial discharge than children with only major depression or dysthymia. Sadly, children hospitalized for depressive disorders had a cumulative risk of rehospitalization after 2 years comparable to children hospitalized with schizophrenia spectrum disorders (Asarnow et al., 1988). Although not yet empirically documented, the impact of such a psychiatric course on normal development and later adult functioning is potentially devastating because of the proportion of "sick time" and the severity of disturbance during important maturational phases.

## *Familial Risk*

In children and adolescents with dysthymia, the preponderance of secondary major depressive and anxiety disorders across inpatient, clinic-referred, and epidemiologic samples suggests a vulnerability to affective-spectrum disorders (Asarnow et al., 1988; Kovacs et al., 1994; Lewinsohn et al., 1991). Indeed, the work of Klein and colleagues (Klein, Taylor, Dickstein, & Harding, 1988a; Klein, Taylor, Dickstein, & Harding, 1988b) provides partial support for familial risk of dysthymia and other affective disorders. Examining the offspring of parents with Research Diagnostic Criteria-defined unipolar major depressive disorder, these investigators found significantly higher rates of dysthymia and major depression in the offspring of depressed parents than in the offspring of chronically ill or normal control parents. Research on the family history of probands with dysthymia also suggests a familial vulnerability for affective disorders associated with childhood onset. For instance, Klein and his group have reported higher rates of unipolar and bipolar disorders in first-degree relatives of early-onset dysthymic adults as compared to adults with late-onset dysthymia or major depression (Klein et al., 1988a, 1988b).

## *Symptomatology*

When compared to major depression, dysthymia in the Pittsburgh cohort was distinguished by the generally low rates of neurovegetative symptoms and the virtual absence of anhedonia and social withdrawal. Dysthymia was characterized primarily by various manifestations of affect dysregulation, including feelings of sadness, feeling unloved and forlorn, irritability, anger, and temper tantrums. The other prominent feature was the cognitive symptom of poor self-esteem. These findings are consistent with the primarily psychological description by Akiskal and colleagues (Akiskal, 1983; Akiskal, Bitar, Puzantian, Rosenthal, Walker, 1978; Akiskal et al., 1980) of symptomatology in patients with chronic depression.

We also found that disobedience was a frequently occurring associated feature of dysthymia. From a clinical perspective, disobedience in connection with a mood disorder in childhood appears to reflect behavioral dysregulation secondary to the dysregulated affect. That is, a youngster with dysthymia might respond in a negative fashion to requests for behavioral conformity because he or she is feeling upset, irritable, and angry. Possibly, this associated feature of dysthymia may partly account for the earlier notion of "masked depression," in which nonaffective symptomatology, such as aggressive acting out, hyperactivity, or psychosomatic complaints, is seen as a defensive response to depression (Cytryn & McKnew, 1972). In contrast, we view acting out in children with dysthymia as the result of an inability to regulate their mood and the subsequent conflict with parents or others when demands are made for compliance or conformity.

## Prevalence

Most of the data regarding the prevalence of dysthymia in juveniles were generated from studies in which DSM-III criteria were used. The rates that have been reported vary, partly owing to across-study differences in sample size, diagnostic criteria, restrictiveness of case definitions, and number of informants. In general, lower rates tend to be reported as a function of large versus small samples, use of DSM-III-R (American Psychiatric Association, 1987) versus DSM-III criteria, stricter definitions of dysthymia, and single versus multiple informants. Table 2.2 (which groups studies according to whether DSM-III or DSM-III-R criteria were used) summarizes the epidemiologic studies of depression in juveniles that provide information specifically about rates of dysthymia.

The rate of DSM-III-defined dysthymia in 7- to 11-year-old

**TABLE 2.2. Epidemiologic Studies of Dysthymic Disorder in Children and Adolescents**

| Study | Year(s) of sampling | Source of information | Prevalence rates (%) | Sample population (age in years) |
|---|---|---|---|---|
| | | DSM-III criteria | | |
| Kashani et al. (1987) | Not reported | Child, parent | 8.0 PP | School (14–16) |
| Costello (1989) | Not reported | Child, parent | 1.3 YP | Pediatric outpatient (7–11) |
| Whitaker et al. (1990) | 1984–1985 | Child | 4.9 LP | School (14–17) |
| McGee et al. (1990) | 1987–1988 | Child, parent | 1.1 YP | Community (15) |
| Garrison, Addy, Jackson, McKeown, & Waller (1992) | 1986–1988 | Child, parent | 8.0 Males, PP<br>5.0 Females, PP | School (12–15) |
| Polaino-Lorente & Domenech (1993) | 1985 | Child | 6.4 PP | School (8–11) |
| | | DSM-III-R criteria | | |
| Lewinsohn, Hops, Roberts, Seeley, & Andrews (1993) | 1987–1989 | Child | 3.2 LP<br>0.5 PP | School (14–18) |
| Fergusson, Horwood, & Lynskey (1993) | 1992 | Child | 0.4 PP | Community (15) |

*Note.* LP, lifetime prevalence; YP, 12-month prevalence; PP, point prevalence.

children ranges from a 12-month prevalence of 1.3% (Costello, 1989) to a point prevalence of 6.4% (Polaino-Lorente & Domenech, 1993). The 6.4% figure, however, is almost certainly an overestimate because caseness was defined only by symptoms and without respect to the required duration of 12 months. Costello's 1.3% rate, based on full diagnostic criteria, including duration, appears to be consistent with the generally low base rates of dysthymia in adolescents. However, the 1.3% figure was derived from a primary care outpatient sample, rather than a community- or school-based sample, and therefore it is unclear whether this rate is representative of the general population. Low rates in children are further suggested by a finding that the combined 12-month prevalence of dysthymia and major depression was 1.8% in 11-year-olds (Anderson, Williams, McGee, & Silva, 1987).

Among adolescents the point prevalence of DSM-III-defined dysthymia has been reported to be 8% (Garrison et al., 1992; Kashani et al., 1987), the 12-month prevalence to be 1.1% (McGee et al., 1990), and the lifetime prevalence by age 17 to be 4.9% (Whitaker et al., 1990). The estimates of point prevalence are probably inflated in comparison to actual population rates. One estimate is based on a sample of 150 adolescents (Kashani et al., 1987); another is from a study in which symptoms were counted toward a diagnosis if they were endorsed by either the parent or the adolescent (Garrison et al., 1992). In the latter study the rate of dysthymia was approximately 3.4% when only symptoms reported by the adolescents were used to determine diagnosis. Nevertheless, this estimate of point prevalence still appears excessive in light of the 1.1% 12-month and 4.9% lifetime prevalence reported by other investigators (McGee et al., 1990; Whitaker et al., 1990). These aforementioned estimates of 12-month and lifetime prevalence, unlike the data for point prevalence, were derived from large community- and school-based samples *and* were based on strict definitions of dysthymia.

According to more recent epidemiologic studies of dysthymia, in which DSM-III-R criteria were used, by age 18 approximately 3% of youths appear to have had DSM-III-R dysthymia (Lewinsohn, Hops, Roberts, Seeley & Andrews, 1993), with a point prevalence among adolescents ranging from 0.4% (Fergusson, Horwood, & Lynskey, 1993) to 0.53% (Lewinsohn et al., 1993). The fact that both studies arrived at a similar estimate of point prevalence and used large samples and strict criteria suggests that these are robust findings. However, prevalence rates from studies using DSM-III-R criteria are not readily comparable to those from studies using DSM-III criteria. DSM-III-R criteria require 2 out of 6 possible symptoms in addition to dysphoric mood, as compared to 3 out of 13 symptoms for DSM-III. Overall, the use of DSM-III-R in epidemiologic studies appears to result in lower prevalence estimates of dysthymia in youths.

In general, therefore, approximately 5% of the population appears to have had DSM-III dysthymia by the end of adolescence, and approximately 1% of children and adolescents may have the disorder during any 12-month period. However, relatively few epidemiologic studies have been conducted. Moreover, many of the studies contain methodological features that obfuscate or may skew estimated rates of dysthymia. For instance, researchers have either combined the categories of major depressive and dysthymic disorders (Anderson et al., 1987; Bird et al., 1988) or age groups (Bird et al., 1988), used samples of uncertain representativeness (Costello, 1989), not used full diagnostic criteria (Polaino-Lorente & Domenech, 1993), or used loose definitions for dysthymia (Garrison et al., 1992). Therefore, the findings must be interpreted cautiously.

An issue of particular interest to the clinician is the proportion of children seen in mental health settings who present with dysthymia. Unfortunately, we are aware of no data other than those from the Pittsburgh Longitudinal Study that bear directly on this issue. In the initial Pittsburgh cohort of 75 consecutive admissions (of children ages 8 to 13 years), only 16% had an initial diagnosis of dysthymia (with or without comorbid major depression). Thus, dysthymia may not be a very common problem in 8- to 13-year-old children seen in child guidance clinics.

## Future Research and Treatment Considerations

Research on very early-onset dysthymic disorder is only in its initial stages. In part, this is due to the relatively recent formal nosological standing of the disorder. It has also long been the case that research in child psychiatry has lagged behind that in adult psychiatry. Thus, further information is needed to clarify three issues regarding dysthymia in general and very early onset dysthymia in particular: First, diagnostic criteria for the disorder continue to change with each new version of the DSM, and there remains some disagreement as to valid criteria (American Psychiatric Association, 1994; Kocsis & Frances, 1987). Second, prospective, long-term follow-ups of juveniles with dysthymia are necessary to further characterize prognosis during childhood and adolescence, as well as outcomes in adults with very early onset. Additional research also is needed to more precisely establish rates of dysthymia in youths. Third, studies are needed to identify efficacious treatments for dysthymia and to determine possible prophylactic effects of early treatment on the subsequent course of the disorder.

In the past three versions of the DSM, there are two different sets of criteria for dysthymic disorder (American Psychiatric Association, 1980, 1987, 1994). Although symptom criteria for diagnosis are unchanged from DSM-III-R to DSM-IV, the latter includes a set of alternative criteria for dysthymic disorder that are analogous to those in DSM-III. The inclusion of alternative criteria in DSM-IV, which are based on a preliminary field trial for this latest version of the manual, is an explicit acknowledgment of the controversy regarding the optimal defining set of symptoms for the diagnosis. Data from the Pittsburgh cohort suggest that the DSM-IV alternative criteria for dysthymia may be more appropriate for juveniles than are the criteria in DSM-III-R or DSM-IV. DSM-IV alternative criteria exclude neurovegetative symptoms, such as sleep and appetite disturbances, and include additional manifestations of affect dysregulation, such as excessive anger. Both of these changes more accurately reflect the relative rates of symptoms in children with dysthymia (Kovacs et al., 1994). Similarly, other investigators have reported that cognitive symptoms and functional difficulties, such as decreased productivity, are more characteristic of dysthymia in adults than neurovegetative symptoms (Kocsis & Frances, 1987).

One pragmatic consideration regarding the different sets of criteria is the relative restrictiveness of each set. A comparison of the DSM-III and DSM-III-R criteria indicates that when DSM-III-R criteria were used, 37.8% fewer prepubertal children with dysthymia were identified than when DSM-III criteria were used (Lahey et al., 1990). All of the dysthymic children identified using DSM-III-R also met DSM-III criteria, suggesting that DSM-III-R is more restrictive. This conclusion is supported when one considers the epidemiologic findings based on the different DSM versions and the consistently lower base rates of dysthymia found using DSM-III-R (e.g., Lewinsohn et al., 1993; Whitaker et al., 1990). Because of the similarity between DSM-III and DSM-IV alternative criteria for dysthymia, one might expect to find roughly equivalent rates using these two different versions; this hypothesis remains to be tested.

Research on dysthymia in juveniles has yet to reach the level of sophistication of work done on major depression. The initial empirical research on major depression in children was conducted to document the phenomenon and was primarily descriptive (e.g., Cytryn & McKnew, 1972; Poznanski & Zrull, 1970; Sandler & Joffe, 1965). Over time, that body of research has become increasingly multifaceted and systematic in identifying symptom criteria, prognosis, family history, biological correlates, and children's responses to antidepressant medication (e.g., Ambrosini, Bianchi, Rabinovich, & Elia, 1993; Rutter et al., 1986; Ryan & Dahl, 1993). It is still the case, however, that descriptions of early-onset dysthymia have been mostly derived from adult samples through retrospective accounts. Additionally, practically nothing is known about the biologic correlates or response to treatment of dysthymic disorder in youths. Juvenile-onset dysthymia therefore requires further study both as a deleterious phenomenon of childhood and as a presumed link to later adult dysfunction and chronic affective disorders.

Large-scale community- or school-based epidemiologic studies of preadolescent samples are needed to determine the actual prevalence of dysthymic disorder in this segment of the population. Such studies must include the use of standardized criteria, such as DSM-IV, and clinically relevant standards for symptom severity and caseness. Two methodological factors that might improve the validity of estimated prevalence rates in preadolescents are reliance on multiple informants and the use of standardized clinical interviews. Multiple informants have been found to result in increased accuracy of diagnosis with preadolescents, particularly regarding depression (Kashani, Orvaschel, Burk, & Reid, 1985; Weissman, Orvaschel, & Padian, 1980).

There is no research of which we are aware that specifically addresses the treatment of dysthymia in juveniles. However, there are varying degrees of evidence for the potential successful treatment of dysthymia in adults by either tricyclic medication or cognitive-behavioral psychotherapy (Akiskal et al., 1980; Kocsis et al., 1988; McCullough, 1991), but controlled clinical trials are needed to replicate these findings. Further research is necessary with tricyclic antidepressants, as there is some evidence that their use by adults with dysthymia may precipitate bipolar episodes (Rihmer et al., 1983). In juveniles, the treatment of depression is an understudied area. There exist few controlled outcome studies of either medication or psychotherapy, particularly with preadolescents. To date, findings from double-blind placebo-controlled studies of antidepressant medication with adolescents and children indicate little difference in response rates to medication and to placebo (Ambrosini et al., 1993). Cognitive and skills-based psychotherapies for depression have been reported to be successful with adolescents, but no consistent effects have been found in controlled trials with preadolescents (Kovacs & Bastiaens, 1995; Weisz, Rudolph, Granger, & Sweeney, 1992). On the basis of preliminary findings with adults, it may be the case that dysthymia in adolescents is responsive to cognitive-behavioral therapy. However, preadolescents remain sorely in need of effective treatments for dysthymia specifically and for depression in general.

Because of subsequent affective comorbidity, early diagnosis of dysthymia in juveniles also may serve to identify individuals at risk for additional affective disorders. Effective early treatment might therefore forestall or lessen the severity of subsequent depressive episodes. Even in cases when early-onset dysthymia is prodromal to a bipolar disorder, early identification might facilitate improved prophylaxis or management. Although very early-onset dysthymia is not a common disorder of childhood, its severity in terms of its protracted duration, lifetime rates of comorbid affective and nonaffective disorders, and presumed impact on adult functioning suggests the necessity of studying the preventive role of early treatment. Interventions would need to include assessment of comorbid conditions and to address them when they are present. Treatment for dysthymia might be directed toward enhancing the child's social and problem-solving skills and might include parent training. The aforementioned goals are suggested by research indicating that depression in children is associated with disruptions in peer and family relations as well as with a negative attributional bias (Armsden, McCauley, Greenberg, Burke, & Mitchell, 1990; Cole & Rehm, 1986; Haley, Fine, Marriage, Moretti, & Freeman, 1985; Puig-Antich et al., 1985). Besides treating the presenting episode, interventions might increase resiliency in youngsters by improving their coping abilities and social support. Parent education might also improve family functioning and serve as an additional buffer against the development of subsequent disorders.

## Conclusion

The available research suggests that dysthymic disorder during childhood and adolescence is a chronic condition. Although dysthymia affects a small proportion of the juvenile population, the severity of the disorder suggests that it warrants greater attention than it has received. The existing research is sparse, and more work is needed to better understand the nature and consequences of dysthymia among our youth. Ultimately, effective treatment of dysthymia among juveniles may have implications for the prevention or amelioration of chronic depression, associated comorbid disorders, and the resulting dysfunction in adulthood.

## Acknowledgment

Preparation of this chapter was supported by Post-Doctoral Fellowship No. 5T32 MH18951 awarded to Andrew G. Renouf and Grant No. MH33990 awarded to Maria Kovacs from the National Institute of Mental Health.

## References

Akiskal, H. S. (1983). Dysthymic disorder: Psychopathology of proposed chronic depressive subtypes. *American Journal of Psychiatry, 140,* 11–20.

Akiskal, H. S. (1991). Chronic depression. *Bulletin of the Menninger Clinic, 55,* 156–171.

Akiskal, H. S., Bitar, A. H., Puzantian, V. R., Rosenthal, T. L., & Walker, P. W. (1978). The nosological status of neurotic depression. A prospective three- to four-year follow-up examination in light of the primary–secondary and unipolar–bipolar dichotomies. *Archives of General Psychiatry, 35,* 756–766.

Akiskal, H. S., Rosenthal, T. L., Haykal, R. F., Lemmi, H., Rosenthal, R. H., & Scott-Strauss, A. (1980). Characterological depressions: Clinical and sleep EEG findings separating "subaffective dysthymias" from "character spectrum disorders." *Archives of General Psychiatry, 37,* 777–783.

Ambrosini, P. J., Bianchi, M. D., Rabinovich, H., & Elia, J. (1993). Antidepressant treatments in children and adolescents: I. Affective disorders. *Journal of the American Academy of Child and Adolescent Psychiatry, 32,* 1–6.

American Psychiatric Association. (1980). *Diagnostic and statistical manual of mental disorders* (3rd ed.). Washington, DC: Author.

American Psychiatric Association. (1987). *Diagnostic and statistical manual of mental disorders* (3rd ed., rev.). Washington, DC: Author.

American Psychiatric Association. (1994). *Diagnostic and statistical manual of mental disorders* (4th ed.). Washington, DC: Author.

Anderson, J. C., Williams, S., McGee, R., & Silva, P. A. (1987). DSM-III disorders in preadolescent children: Prevalence in a large sample from the general population. *Archives of General Psychiatry, 44,* 69–76.

Armsden, G. C., McCauley, E., Greenberg, M. T., Burke, P. M., & Mitchell, J. R. (1990). Parent and peer attachment in early adolescent depression. *Journal of Abnormal Child Psychology, 18,* 683–697.

Asarnow, J. R., Goldstein, M. J., Carlson, G. A., Perdue, S., Bates, S., & Keller, J. (1988). Childhood-onset depressive disorders. *Journal of Affective Disorders, 15,* 245–253.

Bibring, E. (1953). The mechanism of depression. In P. Greenacre (Ed.), *Affective disorders: Psychoanalytic contributions to their study* (pp. 14–47). New York: International Universities Press.

Bird, H. R., Canino, G., Rubio-Stipec, M., Gould, M. S., Ribera, J., Sesman, M., Woodbury, M., Huertas-Goldman, S., Pagan, A., Sanchez-Lacay, A., & Moscoso, M. (1988). Estimates of the prevalence of childhood maladjustment in a community survey in Puerto Rico. *Archives of General Psychiatry, 45,* 1120–1126.

Caron, C., & Rutter, M. (1991). Comorbidity in child psychopathology: Concepts, issues and research strategies. *Journal of Child Psychology and Psychiatry, 32,* 1063–1080.

Cole, D. A., & Rehm, L. P. (1986). Family interaction patterns and childhood depression. *Journal of Abnormal Child Psychology, 14,* 297–314.

Costello, E. J. (1989). Child psychiatric disorders and their correlates: A primary care pediatric sample. *Journal of the American Academy of Child and Adolescent Psychiatry, 28,* 851–855.

Cytryn, L., & McKnew, D. H. (1972). Proposed classification of childhood depression. *American Journal of Psychiatry, 129,* 149–155.

Fergusson, D. M., Horwood, L. J., & Lynskey, M. T. (1993). Prevalence and comorbidity of DSM-III-R diagnoses in a birth cohort of 15 year olds. *Journal of the American Academy of Child and Adolescent Psychiatry, 32,* 1127–1134.

Garrison, C. Z., Addy, C. L., Jackson, K. L., McKeown, R. E., & Waller, J. L. (1992). Major depressive disorder and dysthymia in young adolescents. *American Journal of Epidemiology, 135,* 792–802.

Haley, G. M. T., Fine, S., Marriage, K., Moretti, M. M., & Freeman, R. J. (1985). Cognitive bias and depression in psychiatrically disturbed children and adolescents. *Journal of Consulting and Clinical Psychology, 53,* 535–537.

Kashani, J. H., Carlson, G. A., Beck, N. C., Hoeper, E. W., Corcoran, C.

M., McAllister, J. A., Fallahi, C., Rosenberg, T. K., & Reid, J. C. (1987). Depression, depressive symptoms, and depressed mood among a community sample of adolescents. *American Journal of Psychiatry, 144*, 931–934.

Kashani, J. H., Orvaschel, H., Burk, J. P., & Reid, J. C. (1985). Informant variance: The issue of parent–child disagreement. *Journal of the American Academy of Child Psychiatry, 24*, 437–441.

Keller, M. B., Beardslee, W., Lavori, P. W., Wunder, J., Drs, D. L., & Samuelson, H. (1988). Course of major depression in non-referred adolescents: A retrospective study. *Journal of Affective Disorders, 15*, 235–243.

Keller, M. B., Lavori, P. W., Endicott, J., Coryell, W., & Klerman, G. L. (1983). "Double depression": Two-year follow-up. *American Journal of Psychiatry, 140*, 689–694.

Klein, D. N., Taylor, E. B., Dickstein, S., & Harding, K. (1988a). The early–late onset distinction in DSM-III-R dysthymia. *Journal of Affective Disorders, 14*, 25–33.

Klein, D. N., Taylor, E. B., Dickstein, S., & Harding, K. (1988b). Primary early-onset dysthymia: Comparison with primary nonbipolar non-chronic major depression on demographic, clinical, familial, personality, and socioenvironmental characteristics and short-term outcome. *Journal of Abnormal Psychology, 97*, 387–398.

Klein, D. N., Taylor, E. B., Harding, K., & Dickstein, S. (1990). The unipolar–bipolar distinction in the characterological mood disorders. *Journal of Nervous and Mental Disease, 178*, 318–323.

Kocsis, J. H., & Frances, A. J. (1987). A critical discussion of DSM-III dysthymic disorder. *American Journal of Psychiatry, 144*, 1534–1542.

Kocsis, J. H., Frances, A. J., Voss, C., Mann, J. J., Mason, B. J., & Sweeney, J. (1988). Imipramine treatment for chronic depression. *Archives of General Psychiatry, 45*, 253–257.

Kocsis, J. H., Voss, C., Mann, J. J., & Frances, A. (1986). Chronic depression: Demographic and clinical characteristics. *Psychopharmacology Bulletin, 22*, 192–195.

Kovacs, M. (1985). The Interview Schedule for Children (ISC). *Psychopharmacology Bulletin, 21*, 991–994.

Kovacs, M., Akiskal, H. S., Gatsonis, C., & Parrone, P. L. (1994). Childhood-onset dysthymic disorder: Clinical features and prospective naturalistic outcome. *Archives of General Psychiatry, 51*, 365–374.

Kovacs, M., & Bastiaens, L. J. (1995). The psychotherapeutic management of major depressive and dysthymic disorders in childhood and adolescence: Issues and prospects. In I. M. Goodyer (Ed.), *The depressed child and adolescent: Developmental and clinical perspectives* (pp. 281–310). Cambridge: Cambridge University Press.

Kovacs, M., Feinberg, T. L., Crouse-Novak, M. A., Paulauskas, S. L., & Finkelstein, R. (1984). Depressive disorders in childhood: I. A longitudinal prospective study of characteristics and recovery. *Archives of General Psychiatry, 41*, 229–237.

Kovacs, M., Feinberg, T. L., Crouse-Novak, M., Paulauskas, S. L., Pollock, M., & Finkelstein, R. (1984). Depressive disorders in childhood: II. A longitudinal study of the risk for a subsequent major depression. *Archives of General Psychiatry, 41*, 643–649.

Kovacs, M., & Goldston, D. (1991). Cognitive and social cognitive development of depressed children and adolescents. *Journal of the American Academy of Child and Adolescent Psychiatry, 30*, 388–392.

Lahey, B. B., Loeber, R., Stouthamer-Loeber, M., Christ, M. A. G., Green, S., Russo, M. F., Frick, P. J., & Dulcan, M. (1990). Comparison of DSM-III and DSM-III-R diagnoses for prepubertal children: Changes in prevalence and validity. *Journal of the American Academy of Child and Adolescent Psychiatry, 29*, 620–626.

Lewinsohn, P. M., Hops, H., Roberts, R. E., Seeley, J. R., & Andrews, J. A. (1993). Adolescent psychopathology: I. Prevalence and incidence of depression and other DSM-III-R disorders in high school students. *Journal of Abnormal Psychology, 102*, 133–144.

Lewinsohn, P. M., Rohde, P., Seeley, J. R., & Hops, H. (1991). Comorbidity of unipolar depression: I. Major depression with dysthymia. *Journal of Abnormal Psychology, 100*, 205–213.

McCullough, J. P. (1991). Psychotherapy for dysthymia: A naturalistic study of ten patients. *Journal of Nervous and Mental Disease, 179*, 734–740.

McGee, R., Feehan, M., Williams, S., Partridge, F., Silva, P. A., & Kelly, J. (1990). DSM-III disorders in a large sample of adolescents. *Journal of the American Academy of Child and Adolescent Psychiatry, 29*, 611–619.

Myers, K., McCauley, E., Calderon, R., & Treder, R. (1991). The 3-year longitudinal course of suicidality and predictive factors for subsequent suicidality in youths with major depressive disorder. *Journal of the American Academy of Child and Adolescent Psychiatry, 30*, 804–810.

Polaino-Lorente, A., & Domenech, E. (1993). Prevalence of childhood depression: Results of the first study in Spain. *Journal of Child Psychology and Psychiatry, 34*, 1007–1017.

Poznanski, E., & Zrull, J. P. (1970). Childhood depression. *Archives of General Psychiatry, 23*, 8–15.

Puig-Antich, J. (1980). Affective disorders in childhood. *Psychiatric Clinics of North America, 3*, 403–424.

Puig-Antich, J., Lukens, E., Davies, M., Goetz, D., Brennan-Quattrock, J.,

& Todak, G. (1985). Psychosocial functioning in prepubertal major depressive disorder: I. Interpersonal relationships during the depressive episode. *Archives of General Psychiatry, 42,* 500–527.

Rihmer, Z., Szadoczky, E., & Arato, M. (1983). Dexamethasone suppression test in masked depression. *Journal of Affective Disorders, 5,* 293–296.

Rutter, M., Izard, C. E., & Read, P. B. (Eds.). (1986). *Depression in young people: Developmental and clinical perspectives.* New York: Guilford Press.

Ryan, N. D., & Dahl, R. E. (1993). The biology of depression in children and adolescents. In J. J. Mann & D. J. Kupfer (Eds.), *Biology of depressive disorders, part B: Subtypes of depression and comorbid disorders* (pp. 37–58). New York: Plenum Press.

Sandler, J., & Joffe, W. G. (1965). Notes on childhood depression. *International Journal of Psychoanalysis, 46,* 88–96.

Spitzer, R. L., Endicott, J., & Robins, E. (1978). Research diagnostic criteria: Rationale and reliability. *Archives of General Psychiatry, 35,* 773–782.

Toolan, J. M. (1962). Depression in children and adolescents. *American Journal of Orthopsychiatry, 32,* 404–415.

Warner, V., Weissman, M. M., Fendrich, M., Wickramaratne, P., & Moreau, D. (1992). The course of major depression in the offspring of depressed parents. *Archives of General Psychiatry, 49,* 795–801.

Weissman, M. M., Orvaschel, H., & Padian, N. (1980). Children's symptom and social functioning self-report scales: Comparison of mothers' and children's reports. *Journal of Nervous and Mental Disease, 168,* 736–740.

Weisz, J. R., Rudolph, K. D., Granger, D. A., & Sweeney, L. (1992). Cognition, competence, and coping in child and adolescent depression: Research findings, developmental concerns, therapeutic implications. *Development and Psychopathology, 4,* 627–653.

Whitaker, A., Johnson, J., Shaffer, D., Rapoport, J. L., Kalikow, K., Walsh, B. T., Davies, M., Braiman, S., & Dolinsky, A. (1990). Uncommon troubles in young people: Prevalence estimates of selected psychiatric disorders in a nonreferred adolescent population. *Archives of General Psychiatry, 47,* 487–496.

Winokur, G. (1979). Unipolar depression: Is it divisible into autonomous subtypes? *Archives of General Psychiatry, 36,* 47–52.

Wolfenstein, M. (1966). How is mourning possible? *Psychoanalytic Study of the Child, 21,* 93–123.

CHAPTER THREE

# Comorbidity of Dysthymic Disorder

JOHN C. MARKOWITZ

Research has transformed our understanding of dysthymic disorder in recent years. In the not so distant pre-DSM-III (American Psychiatric Association, 1980) past, chronic depression was considered a "melancholy" character type best treated with psychoanalysis. It is now clear that many patients with dysthymic disorder have mood disorders that respond to antidepressant medications (Kocsis, Frances, Voss, Mann, et al., 1988).

Another clinical maxim once held that chronic depression arises as a nonspecific sequel to other psychiatric and medical disorders. This idea, too, has been contradicted. Dysthymic disorder is indeed strongly associated with comorbid disorders, but there is evidence that most of the dysthymic patients whom psychiatrists see have a primary, rather than a secondary, dysthymia. That is, dysthymic disorder usually comes first and may, on its chronic course, predispose to other disorders. Dysthymic disorder thus does not typically represent a demoralized response to other illness but is a syndrome in its own right. This chapter describes patterns of comorbid disorders associated with dysthymic disorder.

Not only did DSM-III in 1980 bring dysthymic disorder to psychiatry, but its multiaxial system and standardized polythetic diagnoses also ushered in the Age of Comorbidity (Kocsis, Markowitz, & Prien, 1990). Comorbidity has been defined as "any distinct additional clinical entity that has existed or that may occur during the clinical course of a patient who has the index disease under study" (Feinstein, 1970, pp. 456–457). A research industry arose to assess the patterns in which Axis I and Axis II diagnoses co-occurred in psychiatric patients. Does this make comorbidity a dry academic concept? Not necessarily. Some comorbidity studies may prove to be arid exercises for grant monies. In other instances comorbidity may simply reflect overlap of sets of diagnostic criteria for different disorders (Kocsis & Frances, 1987). On the other hand, comorbidity may affect treatment approach and prognosis. For dysthymic disorder, comorbidity appears to be meaningful in some respects, if perhaps not so meaningful in others.

Comorbidity allows us to consider interesting clinical questions: When a dysthymic patient develops panic symptoms, are they symptoms of the mood disorder, symptoms of a discrete anxiety disorder developing from the mood disorder, or symptoms that are independent and coincidental? When a patient with dysthymic disorder of early onset manifests all the features of avoidant personality disorder, has one diagnosis caused the other? Or are depressive symptoms simply masquerading as an avoidant character style? If the latter, effective treatment of dysthymic disorder should eradicate the "personality disorder."

Comorbid diagnoses may disguise dysthymic disorder from clinicians and perhaps may characterize clinically important dysthymic subtypes. Comorbidity itself necessarily defined one subtyping of dysthymia: the distinction made between primary and secondary dysthymia in DSM-III-R (American Psychiatric Association, 1987). We presume—although there are few data to judge—that dysthymic disorder postdating and secondary to a chronic nonmood Axis I or Axis III disorder differs in clinical meaning and potential outcome from the primary type that emerges first and foremost.

Dysthymic disorder and its comorbidity have been studied in two settings: in the general community and among populations of psychiatric patients. This chapter summarizes current knowledge of the comorbidity of dysthymic disorder and attempts to illustrate its clinical relevance and import.

# What Is the Comorbidity of Dysthymic Disorder?

## Comorbidity in the Community

The principal research in this area comes from the Epidemiologic Catchment Area (ECA) Study (Weissman, Leaf, Bruce, & Florio, 1988). The ECA was an ambitious multisite collaborative study of the prevalence and incidence of psychiatric disorders and health care utilization across the United States. Individuals from representative community samples in New Haven, Connecticut, Baltimore, Maryland, St. Louis, Missouri, Piedmont, North Carolina, and Los Angeles, California, were interviewed using the Diagnostic Interview Schedule (DIS) (Regier et al., 1984). A structured interview, the DIS assesses a number of DSM-III diagnoses, including dysthymic disorder but not psychotic, chronic medical, or personality disorders; hence ECA findings do not address comorbidity of dysthymic disorder with Axis II and III disorders. The ECA study found dysthymic disorder in 4% of women, 2% of men, and 3.1% of the overall populace, with prevalence ranging from 2.1% to 4.2% at five sites (Weissman et al., 1988). Weissman and colleagues (1988) found a lifetime comorbidity among dysthymic subjects in the ECA study of 38.9% for major depression, 10.5% for panic disorder, 2.9% for bipolar disorder, 46.2% for any anxiety disorder, 29.8% for substance abuse, and 77.1% for any psychiatric disorder. Dysthymic subjects had an increased risk for having each of these disorders relative to nondysthymics; were more likely to use health and mental health services; and were more likely to receive psychotropic medication, particularly minor tranquilizers.

Dysthymics identified in the ECA study were at increased risk for drug abuse, drug dependence, and alcohol dependence but not for alcohol abuse (Regier et al., 1990). Research on one subsample in St. Louis revealed high comorbidity of dysthymic disorder (7.8 risk ratio) among the 1% of the populace suffering from posttraumatic stress disorder (PTSD) (Helzer, Robins, & McEvoy, 1987). A study of ECA subjects with social phobia likewise uncovered a high comorbidity for dysthymic disorder, with a 4.3 risk ratio (Schneier, Johnson, Hornig, Liebowitz, & Weissman, 1992).

Community sampling by structured clinical interview of 150 adolescents 14 to 16 years old in Columbia, Missouri, diagnosed

12 (8%) as having dysthymic disorder (Kashani et al., 1987). These adolescents met criteria for a significantly greater number of comorbid diagnoses than did their nondysthymic peers. Comorbid diagnoses included anxiety disorder in nine (75%), major depression in seven (58%), oppositional disorder in six (50%), conduct disorder in four (33%), drug (25%) and alcohol (25%) abuse in three apiece, and single diagnoses of mania, attention-deficit disorder, and enuresis.

### Comorbidity among Psychiatric Patients

Comorbidity of dysthymic disorder may differ in the general community and the clinic. In fact, severity of symptoms and degree of comorbidity may define the people in the community who seek treatment and become patients. Studies at the Payne Whitney Clinic (Kocsis et al., 1990; Marin, Kocsis, & Frances, 1992; Markowitz, Moran, Kocsis, & Frances, 1992) and elsewhere (American Psychiatric Association, 1987; Kaufman, 1991; Klein, Taylor, Harding, & Dickstein, 1988; Kovacs, Feinberg, Crouse-Novak, & Richards, 1984; Mezzich, Ahn, Fabrega, & Pilkonis, 1990; Schneier et al., 1992) suggest that dysthymic disorder is prevalent among psychiatric outpatients and rarely appears as an uncomplicated disorder.

## Comorbidity with Axis I Diagnoses

### Major Depression

Major depression is the diagnosis whose overlap with dysthymia has been most closely studied. Keller and colleagues first identified the superimposition of major depression and dysthymic disorder with the rubric of "double depression," noting that doubly depressed patients were less likely to recover during various intervals of follow-up (Keller & Shapiro, 1982). Yet inasmuch as DSM-IV (American Psychiatric Association, 1994) symptom criteria for dysthymic disorder and major depression overlap, with only two additional symptoms needed for the latter, it would seem almost inevitable that dysthymic patients, buffeted by the vicissitudes of a chronically depressed life, would sooner or later develop additional symptoms for the minimum duration of 2 weeks, thus qualifying for major depression and double depression. If so, double depression would simply indicate depressive severity and would constitute an artifactual rather than a true comorbidity (Kocsis & Frances, 1987).

Longitudinal studies of dysthymic patients could answer this question. The only such study to date, by Kovacs and colleagues (Kovacs et al., 1984), indeed found that most in a cohort of dysthymic children and adolescents subsequently developed major depressive episodes. The recent DSM-IV Field Trial on Mood Disorders also found that 79% of 191 subjects meeting criteria for DSM-III-R dysthymia had a lifetime history of major depression (McCullough et al., 1992), again suggesting the strong probability of dysthymic patients ultimately meeting criteria for both diagnoses.

The variation shown in Table 3.1 of percentages of dysthymic patients meeting criteria for major depression doubtless reflects the sampling methods of investigators and the particular populations under study. Klein et al. (1988), for example, sought a sample of double depressives for comparison with patients diagnosed as having major depression without dysthymic disorder.

## Anxiety Disorders

As Table 3.1 indicates, anxiety disorders have been found in roughly half of dysthymic subjects. Given differences in sampling, this proportion shows reasonable stability. Mezzich et al. (1990), who described the largest patient sample and found the lowest point prevalence of anxiety disorders, used an instrument whose sensitivity may differ from other studies. In our study comparing 34 outpatients with Structured Clinical Interview for DSM-III-R (SCID)-diagnosed dysthymia to 56 nondysthymic outpatients, social phobia was significantly more prevalent among dysthymic subjects (Markowitz et al., 1992).

Cloninger and colleagues (Cloninger, Martin, Guze, & Clayton, 1990) asserted that dysthymia typically postdates anxiety disorders, yet most of the studies cited (Markowitz, Moran, Kocsis, & Frances, 1992; Sanderson, Beck, & Beck, 1990), including the only prospective research (Kovacs et al., 1984), found that dysthymic disorder usually comes first and anxiety disorders follow.

**TABLE 3.1. Axis I Comorbidity of Dysthymic Disorder among Psychiatric Patients**

| Study | *n* | Major depression | Anxiety disorder | Substance abuse | Eating disorders | Remarks |
|---|---|---|---|---|---|---|
| Sanderson, Beck, & Beck (1990) | 63 | n/a | 48% | 11% | 0% | SCID |
| Kovacs, Feinberg, & Crouse-Novak (1989) | 39 | 41% | 44% | n/a | n/a | Adolescents; longitudinal |
| Klein, Taylor, Harding, & Dickstein (1988) | 31 | 100% | 71% | 45% | 23% | "Double depressives"; SCID |
| Mezzich, Ahn, Fabrega, & Pilkonis | 261 | 31% | 25% | 14% | n/a | Initial Evaluation Form |
| Markowitz, Moran, Kocsis, & Frances (1992) | 34 | 68% | 68% | 24% | 12% | SCID |

## Substance Abuse and Other Diagnoses

Chronically depressed people may use recreational drugs to self-medicate their mood disorder. Alternatively, dysthymic disorder may reflect the protracted dysphoria some former substance abusers experience during abstinence. Dysthymic disorder must be distinguished from chronic substance-induced affective symptoms induced by active cocaine or other drug use. Whatever the relationship, a significant prevalence of substance abuse has been reported among dysthymic patients in most studies that have examined it (Klein et al., 1988; Kovacs et al., 1984; Markowitz, Moran, Kocsis, & Frances, 1992; Weissman et al., 1988). Eating disorders, known to have a significant association with mood disorder, have also been found in comorbidity studies of dysthymic patients.

Among cohorts of patients primarily identified as having other psychiatric disorders, dysthymic disorder commonly appears as a comorbid condition. For example, Barsky, Wyshak, and Klerman (1992) studied 42 patients with DSM-III-R hypochondriasis and found dysthymia to be their most prevalent comorbid Axis I disorder, affecting 45% of subjects. Devlin and Walsh (1989) reported that 38% of 50 subjects with bulimia, anorexia, or both suffered from Research Diagnostic Criteria (RDC)-diagnosed intermittent depression (roughly corresponding to dysthymic disorder). Halmi and colleagues found that 20% of 62 patients with DSM-III-R anorexia nervosa met criteria for dysthymia, compared to 2% of controls (Halmi et al., 1991). Since all of these disorders have known associations with depression, such findings confirm clinical intuition.

## Comorbidity with Axis II Diagnoses

Various Axis II diagnoses have also been associated with dysthymic disorder (see Table 3.2). The text of DSM-III suggested the possible association of dysthymic disorder with borderline, histrionic, and dependent personality disorders, and DSM-III-R added narcissistic and avoidant personality disorders to the list. Akiskal (1983, p. 17) found "a liberal melange of 'unstable' characterologic treats, with dependent, histrionic, antisocial, or schizoid features" among his character-spectrum subtype of chronic depressives. The chart review by Koenigsberg and colleagues (Koenigsberg, Kaplan, Gilmore, & Cooper, 1985) of 2,462 psychiatric patients revealed that 34% of the 68 dysthymic patients had Axis II comorbidity: 16% were classified mixed–atypical–other; 7%, dependent personality disorder; and 6%, borderline personality disorder. Kocsis and colleagues (Kocsis, Voss, Mann, & Frances, 1986) found that a sample of dysthymic outpatients had a 47% prevalence of personality disorder, with dependent (23%) and atypical–mixed (13%) personality disorders the most frequent Axis II diagnoses. Klein et al. (1988) reported a 48% prevalence of "severe personality disorder," comprising borderline, antisocial, and schizotypal personality disorders.

Sanderson and colleagues (Sanderson, Wetzler, Beck, & Beck, 1992) used the SCID-II to interview 197 patients with major depression alone, 63 patients with pure dysthymia (i.e., uncomplicated by major depression), and 32 patients with double depression. Half of the patients with major depression, 52% of dysthymic patients, and 69% of patients with double depression met criteria for at least one personality disorder. Cluster A diagnoses were rare and cluster C diagnoses most common in both chronically depressed samples.

Our study, which also used the SCID-II to assess outpatients,

## TABLE 3.2. Axis II Comorbidity of Dysthymic Disorder among Psychiatric Patients

| | | | Odd cluster | | | Dramatic cluster | | | | Anxious cluster | | | | | |
|---|---|---|---|---|---|---|---|---|---|---|---|---|---|---|---|
| Study | $n$ | Any | Par | Sz | Sztp | His | Nar | Asoc | Bor | Avd | Dep | Comp | PsAg | S-def | Atyp/mixed |
| Koenigsberg, Kaplan, Gilmore, & Cooper (1985) | 68 | 34% | 0% | 0% | 1% | 1% | 1% | 0% | 6% | 0% | 7% | 0% | 0% | | 16% |
| Kocsis, Voss, Mann, & Frances (1986) | 39 | 47% | | | 8% | | 8% | | | 10% | 23% | 5% | | | 13% |
| Mezzich, Ahn, Fabrega, & Pilkonis (1990) | 139 | 38% | | 5% | | | | 5% | | | | 18% | | | 11% |
| Oldham & Skodol (1991) | 372 | n/a[a] | | 7% | | | 12% | | 28% | | | 52% | | | n/a |
| Sanderson, | 63 | 52%[b] | 3% | 0% | 2% | 2% | 6% | 2% | 8% | 22% | 8% | 13% | 3% | | 6% |
| Wetzler, Beck, & Betz (1992) | 32 | 69%[c] | 0% | 0% | 3% | 0% | 3% | 3% | 16% | 16% | 19% | 9% | 3% | | 9% |
| Markowitz, Moran, Kocsis, & Frances (1992) | 34 | 85% | 3% | 0% | 12% | 12% | 6% | 0% | 24% | 32% | 21% | 6% | 0% | 35% | 18% |

*Note.* Par, paranoid; Sz, schizoid; Sztp, schizotypal; His, histrionic; Nar, narcissistic; Asoc, antisocial; Bor, borderline; Avd, avoidant; Dep, dependent; Comp, obsessive–compulsive; PsAg, passive–aggressive; S-def, self-defeating; Atyp, atypical.

[a]Of dysthymic subjects with chart diagnoses of comorbid personality disorder.

[b]Pure dysthymics.

yielded results similar to those of the Sanderson et al. (1992) study. Outpatients with dysthymic disorder frequently met criteria for personality disorder. They were significantly more likely to meet criteria for self-defeating (35%), avoidant (32%), dependent (21%), and borderline (24%) personality disorders than were nondysthymic outpatients. Dysthymic subjects were also more likely to meet criteria for avoidant and self-defeating personality disorders than were subjects meeting criteria for major depression but without dysthymia (Markowitz, Moran, Kocsis, & Frances, 1992). Two large additional studies corroborated these findings in reporting a predominance of Cluster C ("anxious") personality disorders among dysthymic patients (Mezzich et al., 1990; Oldham & Skodol, 1991).

## Comorbidity with Axis III Diagnoses

Axis III comorbidity has been noted to affect prognosis of acute depression (Popkin, Callies, & MacKenzie, 1985) but has received little study in relation to dysthymic disorder. Medical comorbidity may largely define *secondary* dysthymic disorder, although some patients with primary dysthymic disorder may later develop physical illness. In the differential diagnosis of dysthymic disorder, clinicians must rule out organic mood syndromes due to infection, endocrinopathy, stroke, etc. (DSM-IV makes no distinction regarding the duration of organic mood syndromes, as it does between functional acute major depression and chronic dysthymic disorder.)

The Rand Medical Outcomes Study reported that dysthymic disorder and other depressive disorders are associated with poor physical health and a variety of chronic medical problems (Wells et al., 1989). Our series of consecutive psychiatric outpatient assessments found little Axis III comorbidity (Markowitz, Moran, Kocsis, & Frances, 1992): 5 (15%) of 34 dysthymic subjects had significant Axis III disorders, a rate comparable to nondysthymic subjects. Yet findings might well differ among medical outpatients with dysthymic disorder, depending on the nature of their medical illness. Elevated lifetime rates of dysthymic disorder have been found among patients seeking treatment for insomnia (45% in a study by Tan, Kales, Kales, Soldatos, & Bixler, 1984), but not among morbidly obese (8% in a study by Black, Goldstein, & Mason, 1992) or type I diabetic patients (4% in a study by Popkin, Callies, Lentz, Colon, & Sutherland, 1988).

In summary, dysthymic disorder rarely presents in the absence of other diagnoses. Dysthymic individuals, both in the community and in the clinic, are likely to meet criteria for concomitant major depression in their lifetimes, have roughly a 50% chance of developing an anxiety disorder, and are also at elevated risk for substance abuse and perhaps eating disorders. Dysthymic disorder frequently predates the onset of comorbid Axis I disorders among clinic patients. Axis II diagnoses are also prevalent, particularly from the "anxious" Cluster C. Less research has examined Axis III comorbidity, but dysthymic disorder may be associated with poor physical health.

## Why Is Comorbidity of Dysthymic Disorder Important?

### *Comorbidity May Mask Dysthymic Disorder*

Weissman and Klerman reported in 1977 that chronically depressed patients were often misdiagnosed as primarily suffering from anxiety, were often treated with benzodiazepines rather than antidepressant medications, and often remained depressed at follow-up. This situation had not changed by the mid-1980s, when the ECA study found dysthymic patients to be high utilizers of health care and particularly prone to receiving minor tranquilizers. The trend likely continues today, although one might hope that the increasing trend of general medical practitioners to prescribe selective serotonin reuptake inhibitors indicates a change in this pattern.

Dysthymic disorder tends to evoke despair. Doctors and mental health professionals, dispirited by the chronicity of the patient's mood disorder, may inadvertently focus on anxiety symptoms or comorbid anxiety disorders rather than confront the patient's underlying dysthymic disorder. Clinicians who ignore DSM-IV (American Psychiatric Association, 1994) diagnosis in favor of character pathology may focus on character traits that could be epiphenomena of dysthymic disorder. Such confusion is unfortunate, since vigorous therapy of dysthymic disorder can be highly effective (Kocsis, Frances, Voss, Mann, et al., 1988). We urge clinicians to look for dysthymic disorder beneath its comorbidity and to treat patients with antidepressant medications and/or focused antidepressant psychotherapy (Markowitz, 1994) such as interpersonal therapy (Klerman, Weissman, Rounsaville, & Chevron, 1984; Mason, Markowitz, & Klerman, 1993) or cognitive-behavioral therapy (McCullough, 1991; Mercier, Stewart, & Quitkin, 1992) (see Chapter 9, this volume).

## Comorbidity May Affect Treatment Outcome of Dysthymic Disorder

Comorbidity may influence the treatment of dysthymic disorder in several respects. Clusters of comorbid diagnoses might predict response to pharmacological and psychotherapeutic treatments. It would be useful to know, for example, whether comorbid social phobia predicts a robust pharmacological response for dysthymic disorder or whether presence of schizotypal personality disorder or multiple sclerosis worsens prognosis. A variety of studies suggest comorbidity may influence treatment outcome for patients with major depression (e.g., Grunhaus, 1988; Shea et al., 1990); how and whether this applies to dysthymic disorder is less clear.

In some studies (Keller & Shapiro, 1982; Klein et al., 1988), patients with double depression were less likely than pure dysthymics to respond to treatment, but this might be explained by low medication doses in naturalistic follow-ups or by the fact that greater *severity* of symptoms among double depressives requires greater improvement to reach remission. Marin and colleagues (1992) found that although no single comorbid diagnosis—including double depression—alone compromised acute treatment outcome, dysthymic patients who had comorbid diagnoses were overall more likely to partially respond (odds ratio = 1.8) than fully respond (odds ratio = 0.70) to desipramine. Preliminary analysis of 97 dysthymic patients treated by Kocsis and colleagues with 10 weeks of desipramine revealed no effect of double depression, of comorbid Axis I anxiety disorders, or of comorbid Axis II "anxious" (Cluster C) personality disorders on outcome relative to pure dysthymia (Lewinter, Kocsis, & Markowitz, 1993).

## Treatment Outcome May Affect Comorbidity of Dysthymic Disorder

Anxiety symptoms appear on the Hamilton Rating Scale for Depression (HRSD) and have long been recognized as symptoms of depression. Clinicians intuitively appreciate the depressive nature of dependent, avoidant, and masochistic personality traits. Dysthymic disorder is so pervasive and so chronic that it affects most aspects of a patient's life. It may trespass on other diagnostic criteria sets and mimic other disorders—an artifactual comorbidity—or it may give rise or predispose to discrete anxiety disorders and other conditions. In either case, remission of dysthymic disorder may be accompanied by improvement in comorbid disorders. Such improvement in comorbid diagnoses has been noted in treating obsessive–compulsive disorder as well (Ricciardi et al., 1992).

Axis II diagnoses, particularly avoidant, dependent, and self-defeating personality disorders, with their affectively tinged behaviors, may reflect the effects of chronically depressed mood on personality. When a "state" condition such as a depressive episode is lifelong, how can it be distinguished from a "trait"? This is indeed a significant clinical problem for dysthymic patients, who tend to see their mood disorder as their personality. Because of this difficulty in distinguishing state from trait in the presence of chronic mood disorder, the clinician should avoid prejudging patients as character disordered until the depression has lifted (Bronisch & Klerman, 1991; Markowitz, 1993a).

Being depressed all one's life can deform self-image and interpersonal behaviors. In our experience, successful treatment of dysthymic disorder not only improves social and vocational functioning (Kocsis, Frances, Voss, Mason, et al., 1988; Markowitz, Moran, & Kocsis, 1992; Stewart et al., 1988) but also can seemingly change character. Maladaptive traits resulting from dysthymic disorder may resolve or transform when the mood disorder is effectively treated (Bronisch & Klerman, 1991). It is therefore important for the psychotherapist not to assume that character in dysthymic patients is static but to reserve judgment until after the weight of depressed mood has been lifted.

This area of chronic "state" masquerading as "trait" has thus far received little study. I here report two cases of patients with pure DSM-III-R dysthymia of early primary onset who presented for treatment with interpersonal therapy (Mason et al., 1993). One, a 27-year-old married white woman, met criteria for comorbid borderline and dependent personality disorder on a structured interview; the other, a 44-year-old married white woman, qualified for borderline and self-defeating personality disorders. Both reported virtually lifelong depressive symptoms. At the end of 16 weekly sessions, their mean HRSD scores had fallen from 16.0 at baseline to 6.5. When reassessed by SCID-P and SCID-II, they met criteria neither for dysthymia nor for the comorbid personality disorders. Recovery from dysthymia made them feel stronger and more competent, and life's pressures seemed less overwhelming and anxiety provoking to them than before. Both have maintained their improvement at 1-year (and one at 2-year) follow-up.

## Conclusion

Siamese sibling offspring of DSM-III, dysthymic disorder and comorbidity have shared destinies. Dysthymic disorder has been more closely associated with comorbid conditions than have most other disorders, although received ideas of what this relationship means have been undercut by recent research. Rather than representing secondary demoralization from other disorders, dysthymic disorder often appears as a primary demoralization for patients; it is a pervasive, lingering disorder that may predispose to the onset of major depression, anxiety disorders, and other conditions. Comorbidity should continue to play an important role in the recognition and treatment of dysthymic disorder. Clinicians who ignore it do so at their peril.

## Acknowledgment

This chapter is adapted from Markowitz (1993b). Copyright 1993 by Slack, Inc. Adapted by permission.

## References

Akiskal, H. S. (1983). Dysthymic disorder: Psychopathology of proposed chronic depressive subtypes. *American Journal of Psychiatry, 140,* 11–20.

American Psychiatric Association. (1980). *Diagnostic and statistical manual of mental disorders* (3rd ed.). Washington, DC: Author.

American Psychiatric Association. (1987). *Diagnostic and statistical manual of mental disorders* (3rd ed., rev.). Washington, DC: Author.

American Psychiatric Association. (1994). *Diagnostic and statistical manual of mental disorders* (4th ed.). Washington, DC: Author.

Barsky, A. J., Wyshak, G., & Klerman, G. L. (1992). Psychiatric comorbidity in DSM-III-R hypochondriasis. *Archives of General Psychiatry, 49*, 101–108.

Black, D. W., Goldstein, R. B., & Mason, E. E. (1992). Prevalence of mental disorder in 88 morbidly obese bariatric clinic patients. *American Journal of Psychiatry, 149*, 227–234.

Bronisch, T., & Klerman, G. L. (1991). Personality functioning: Change and stability in relationship to symptoms and psychopathology. *Journal of Personality Disorders, 5*, 307–317.

Cloninger, C. R., Martin, R. L., Guze, S. B., & Clayton, P. J. (1990). The empirical structure of psychiatric comorbidity and its theoretical significance. In J. D. Maser & C. R. Cloninger (Eds.), *Comorbidity of mood and anxiety disorders* (pp. 439–462). Washington, DC: American Psychiatric Press.

Devlin, M. J., & Walsh, B. T. (1989). Eating disorders and depression. *Psychiatric Annals, 19*, 473–476.

Feinstein, A. R. (1970). The pre-therapeutic classification of comorbidity in chronic disease. *Journal of Chronic Diseases, 23*, 455–468.

Grunhaus, L. (1988). Clinical and psychobiological characteristics of simultaneous panic disorder and major depression. *American Journal of Psychiatry, 145*, 1214–1221.

Halmi, K. A., Eckert, E., Marchi, P., Sampugnaro, V., Apple, R., & Cohen, J. (1991). Comorbidity of psychiatric diagnoses in anorexia nervosa. *Archives of General Psychiatry, 48*, 712–718.

Helzer, J. E., Robins, L. N., & McEvoy, L. (1987). Post-traumatic stress disorder in the general population. *New England Journal of Medicine, 317*, 1630–1634.

Kashani, J. H., Carlson, G. A., Beck, N. C., Hoeper, E. W., Corcoran, C. M., McAllister, J. A., Fallahi, C., Rosenberg, T. K., & Reid, J. C. (1987). Depression, depressive symptoms, and depressed mood among a community sample of adolescents. *American Journal of Psychiatry, 144*, 931–934.

Kaufman, J. (1991). Depressive disorders in maltreated children. *Journal of the American Academy of Child and Adolescent Psychiatry, 30*(2), 257–265.

Keller, M. B., & Shapiro, R. W. (1982). "Double depression": Superimposition of acute depressive episodes on chronic depressive disorders. *American Journal of Psychiatry, 139*, 438–442.

Klein, D. N., Taylor, E. B., Harding, K., & Dickstein, S. (1988). Double depression and episodic major depression: Demographic, clinical, familial, personality, and socioenvironmental characteristics and short-term outcome. *American Journal of Psychiatry, 145*, 1226–1231.

Klerman, G. L., Weissman, M. M., Rounsaville, B. J., & Chevron, E. S. (1984). *Interpersonal psychotherapy of depression.* New York: Basic Books.

Kocsis, J. H., & Frances, A. J. (1987). A critical discussion of DSM-III dysthymic disorder. *American Journal of Psychiatry, 144*, 1534–1542.

Kocsis, J. H., Frances, A. J., Voss, C., Mann, J. J., Mason, B. J., & Sweeney, J. (1988). Imipramine treatment for chronic depression. *Archives of General Psychiatry, 45*, 253–257.

Kocsis, J. H., Frances, A. J., Voss, C., Mason, B. J., Mann, J. J., & Sweeney, J. (1988). Imipramine and social-vocational adjustment in chronic depression. *American Journal of Psychiatry, 145*, 997–999.

Kocsis, J. H., Markowitz, J. C., & Prien, R. F. (1990). Comorbidity of dysthymic disorder. In C. R. Cloninger (Ed.), *Comorbidity in anxiety and mood disorders* (pp. 317–328). Washington, DC: American Psychiatric Press.

Kocsis, J. H., Voss, C., Mann, J. J., & Frances, A. (1986). Chronic depression: Demographic and clinical characteristics. *Psychopharmacology Bulletin, 22*, 192–195.

Koenigsberg, H. W., Kaplan, R. D., Gilmore, M. M., & Cooper, A. M. (1985). The relationship between syndrome and personality disorder in DSM-III: Experience with 2,462 patients. *American Journal of Psychiatry, 142*, 207–212.

Kovacs, M., Feinberg, T. L., Crouse-Novak, M. A., & Richards, M. A. (1984). Depressive disorders in childhood: I. A longitudinal prospective study of characteristics and recovery. *Archives of General Psychiatry, 41*, 229–237.

Lewinter, D., Kocsis, J., & Markowitz, J. (1993). *Dysthymia and anxiety: The impact of comorbidity on antidepressant treatment response.* Unpublished manuscript.

Marin, D. B., Kocsis, J. H., & Frances, A. J. (1992, May). *Comorbidity and treatment outcome of dysthymia.* Paper presented at the annual meeting of the American Psychiatric Association, Washington, DC.

Markowitz, J. C. (1993a). Psychotherapy of the post-dysthymic patient. *Journal of Psychotherapy Practice and Research, 2*, 157–163.

Markowitz, J. C. (1993b). Comorbidity of dysthymia. *Psychiatric Annals, 23*(11), 617–624.

Markowitz, J. C. (1994). Psychotherapy of dysthymia. *American Journal of Psychiatry, 151*, 1114–1121.

Markowitz, J. C., Moran, & M. E., Kocsis, J. H. (1992, May). *Response of dysthymic interpersonal deficits to desipramine treatment.* Paper presented at the annual meeting of the New Clinical Drug Evaluation Unit, Boca Raton, FL.

Markowitz, J. C., Moran, M. E., Kocsis, J. H., & Frances, A. J. (1992). Prevalence and comorbidity of dysthymic disorder. *Journal of Affective Disorders, 24*, 63–71.

Mason, B. J., Markowitz, J. C., & Klerman, G. L. (1993). IPT for dysthymic disorder. In G. L. Klerman & M. M. Weissman (Eds.), *New applications of interpersonal therapy* (pp. 225–264). Washington, DC: American Psychiatric Press.

McCullough, J. P. (1991). Psychotherapy for dysthymia: A naturalistic study of ten patients. *Journal of Nervous and Mental Disease, 179*, 734–740.

McCullough, J. P., Klein, D. N., Shea, M. T., et al. (1992, September). *DSM-IV Field Trial for Major Depression, Dysthymia, and Minor Depression.* Abstracts of the annual meeting of the American Psychological Association, Washington, DC.

Mercier, M. A., Stewart, J. W., & Quitkin, F. M. (1992). A pilot sequential study of cognitive therapy and pharmacotherapy of atypical depression. *Journal of Clinical Psychiatry, 53*, 166–170.

Mezzich, J. E., Ahn, C. W., Fabrega, H., & Pilkonis, P. A. (1990). Patterns of psychiatric comorbidity in a large population presenting for care. In J. D. Maser & C. R. Cloninger (Eds.), *Comorbidity in anxiety and mood disorders* (pp. 189–204). Washington, DC: American Psychiatric Press.

Oldham, J. M., & Skodol, A.E. (1991). Personality disorders in the public sector. *Hospital and Community Psychiatry, 42*, 481–487.

Popkin, M. K., Callies, A. L., Lentz, R. D., Colon, E. A., & Sutherland, D. E. (1988). Prevalence of major depression, simple phobia, and other psychiatric disorders in patients with long-standing type I diabetes mellitus. *Archives of General Psychiatry, 45*, 64–68.

Popkin, M. K., Callies, A. L., & Mackenzie, T. B. (1985). The outcome of antidepressant use in the medically ill. *Archives of General Psychiatry, 42*, 1160–1163.

Regier, D. A., Farmer, M. E., Rae, D. S., Locke, B. Z., Keith, S. J., Judd, L. L., & Goodwin, F. K. (1990). Comorbidity of mental disorders with alcohol and other drug abuse. *Journal of the American Medical Association, 264*, 2511–2518.

Regier, D. A., Myers, J. K., Kramer, M., Robins, L. N., Blazer, D. G., Hough, R. L., Eaton, W. W., & Locke, B. Z. (1984). The NIMH Epidemiologic Catchment Area program: Historical context, major objectives, and study population characteristics. *Archives of General Psychiatry, 41*, 934–941.

Ricciardi, J. N., Baer, L., Jenike, M. A., Fischer, S. C., Sholtz, D., & Buttolph, M. L. (1992). Changes in DSM-III-R Axis II diagnoses following treatment of obsessive-compulsive disorder. *American Journal of Psychiatry, 149*, 829–831.

Sanderson, W. C., Beck, A. T., & Beck, J. (1990). Syndrome comorbidity in patients with major depression or dysthymia: Prevalence and temporal relationships. *American Journal of Psychiatry, 147*, 1025–1028.

Sanderson, W. C., Wetzler, S., Beck, A. T., & Betz, F. (1992). Prevalence of personality disorders in patients with major depression and dysthymia. *Psychiatry Research, 42*, 93–99.

Schneier, F. R., Johnson, J., Hornig, C. D., Liebowitz, M. R., & Weissman, M. M. (1992). Social phobia: Comorbidity and morbidity in an epidemiologic sample. *Archives of General Psychiatry, 49*, 282–288.

Shea, M. T., Pilkonis, P. A., Beckham, E., Collins, J. F., Elkin, I., Sotsky, S. M., & Docherty, J. P. (1990). Personality disorders and treatment outcome in the NIMH Treatment of Depression Collaborative Research Program. *American Journal of Psychiatry, 147*, 711–718.

Stewart, J. W., Quitkin, F. M., McGrath, P. J., Rabkin, J. G., Markowitz, J. S., Tricamo, E., & Klein, D. F. (1988). Social functioning in chronic depression: Effect of 6 weeks of antidepressant treatment. *Psychiatric Research, 25*, 213–222.

Tan, T.-L., Kales, J. D., Kales, A., Soldatos, C. R., & Bixler, E. O. (1984). Biopsychobehavioral correlates of insomnia: IV. Diagnosis based on DSM-III. *American Journal of Psychiatry, 141*, 357–362.

Weissman, M. M., & Klerman, G. L. (1977). The chronic depressive in the community: Underrecognized and poorly treated. *Comprehensive Psychiatry, 18*, 523–531.

Weissman, M. M., Leaf, P. J., Bruce, M. L., & Florio, L. (1988). The epidemiology of dysthymia in five communities: Rates, risks, comorbidity, and treatment. *American Journal of Psychiatry, 145*, 815–819.

Wells, K. B., Stewart, A., Hays, R. D., Burnam, M. A., Rogers, W., Daniels, M., Berry, S., Greenfield, S., & Ware, J. (1989). The functioning and well-being of depressed patients. *Journal of the American Medical Association, 262*, 914–919.

CHAPTER FOUR

# Course and Natural History of Chronic Depression

MARTIN B. KELLER
DIANE L. HANKS

Depression is one of the most common of the major psychiatric disorders. The Epidemiologic Catchment Area Study reports an 8% lifetime prevalence for depression in the general population. Table 4.1 presents prevalence data for separate but related forms of depression and indicates that the lifetime probability of someone experiencing an episode of unipolar depression is approximately 5%, of bipolar disorder approximately 1%, and of dysthymia approximately 3% (Regier et al., 1988).

During the last decade, researchers and clinicians have become increasingly aware that major depression, which was once thought to consist of discrete episodes of illness followed by full recovery, is both chronic and recurrent in many patients. Research and clinical observations have shown that patients with depression have a significant likelihood of experiencing relapse, recurrence, chronicity, and residual subsyndromal symptoms in the interval between full criteria episodes of illness (Keller, 1985).

In this chapter the course and natural history of chronic depression is described and its definition expanded to differentiate chronic major depression, dysthymia, and double depression. Chronic major depression can be diagnosed when full criteria for a major depressive episode have been met continuously for at least the past 2 years. Dysthymia is characterized by a chronic depressed

**TABLE 4.1. Prevalence of Depressive Disorders**

| Disorder | Lifetime (%) | Current (%) |
|---|---|---|
| Major depressive episode | | |
| Any episode | 6 | 2.2 |
| Unipolar only | 5 | 1.8 |
| Bipolar | 1 | 0.4 |
| Dysthymia[a] | 3 | 1.6 |
| Any affective disorder | 8 | 5.1 |

*Note.* From Keller (1994). Copyright 1994 by Munksgaard International Publishers, Ltd. Reprinted by permission.

[a]Double depression was diagnosed in 25% of subjects within the 6 months preceding the study; 50% had a lifetime diagnosis of double depression.

mood that is present more days than not for at least 2 years but with symptoms less severe than those of major depressive disorder (American Psychiatric Association, 1994). Double depression is a term used to describe a condition in which a person is suffering from a major depressive episode and also has a chronic minor depression that has preceded the major depression by a duration of at least 2 years. In cases where dysthymia follows directly after a major depression, the diagnosis is major depression in partial remission. If there has been a full remission from a major depressive episode for at least 6 months before the development of dysthymia, then dysthymia can be diagnosed (Keller & Russell, in press). It has been demonstrated that these distinctions, although complex, are related to differences in course, including time to recovery and rates of relapse (Keller & Lavori, 1984; Keller, Lavori, Endicott, Coryell, & Klerman, 1983; Klein, Taylor, Harding, & Dickstein, 1988).

The chapter discusses recent data on course, chronicity, recurrence, relapse, and predictors of outcome in patients suffering from chronic depression, dysthymia, and double depression. Many of the data come from the National Institute of Mental Health (NIMH) Collaborative Depression Study (CDS), a prospective, naturalistic study of over 955 depressed patients who sought treatment at one of five study sites nationwide: Boston (Massachusetts General Hospital, Massachusetts Mental Health Center, Brockton Veterans Affairs Hospital), Chicago (Rush Medical College), Iowa City (Department of Psychiatry, University of Iowa School of Medicine), New York City (New York State Psychiatric Institute), and St. Louis (Department of Psychiatry, Washington

University School of Medicine). In addition, recent data from the DSM-IV (American Psychiatric Association, 1994) Mood Disorders Field Trial, which was designed to assess the relationship between major depression, dysthymia, minor depression, and depressive personality disorder, is presented here.

## Collaborative Depression Study: Evidence of Chronicity

Evidence that depression is a chronic condition has consistently emerged from the CDS since its inception in 1974. At each interval of follow-up the data have suggested that a significant percentage of patients remain chronically ill despite the widely held clinical belief that depressed patients tend to make complete recoveries from acute depressive episodes.

In the CDS, chronic depression referred to a depressive disorder that met the Research Diagnostic Criteria (RDC) for a diagnosis of major depressive disorder, intermittent depressive disorder, or minor depressive disorder of 2 years duration or longer. In order to be considered recovered from a chronic depressive disorder, the patient has to be recovered from the major depressive disorder and has to be completely free of the criterion symptoms for minor or intermittent depressive disorder for 8 consecutive weeks (Keller & Shapiro, 1982).

A 5-year prospective follow-up study of 431 CDS subjects showed that approximately 70% of the patients recovered from their major depressive episode in 1 year. After 2 years the cumulative probability of recovery was 81%, after 4 years 87%, and after 5 years 88% (Keller et al., 1992). After 8 years 7% of the subjects still had not recovered. Probabilities were calculated for intervals ranging from 1 week to 5 years and showed that the chances of recovery from major depression were best within the first 6 months following entry into the study. The longer subjects were depressed, the less likely recovery became, as suggested by the fact that only 18% of the probands still depressed after 1 year of follow-up recovered during the interval between the first and fifth years whereas 54% recovered during the first 6 months after enrollment in the study. The majority of patients who did not recover during the 5 years of follow-up experienced subcriteria symptoms of depression most of the time. Their illness resembled chronic minor depression or dysthymia with superimposed episodes of major depression rather than major depression alone (Keller et al., 1992).

## Double Depression

Studies have found that a substantial number of patients with major depression suffer from a preexisting chronic minor depressive condition such as dysthymia (Keller & Shapiro, 1982). In cases such as these a diagnosis of double depression has been used to depict the coexistence of both disorders (Keller & Lavori, 1984). Recognizing the presence of double depression is important for clinical practice and research, because it greatly influences our measurement of recovery rates, time to relapse following recovery, and predictors of these outcomes in patients who have a major depression. In addition, it has also been shown that patients with double depression experience more severe symptoms and greater comorbidity than do patients with episodic major depression (Klein et al., 1988).

Eighty (25%) of the first 316 patients who entered the CDS with an episode of major depressive disorder had a preexisting chronic depression that had lasted for at least 2 years before the onset of the major depression (Keller et al., 1983). Analysis of the duration of chronic depression prior to intake indicated that 96% of the "double depressed" patients had chronic minor depression lasting 3 years or more, 73% had been ill for 5 years or more, and 42% had been ill for 10 years or more. There was a significantly higher recovery rate at 2 years from the major depression for patients with a double depression (97%) than for patients with a major depression alone (79%) (see Table 4.2). Further analysis revealed that people with double depression did not become as healthy upon recovery as those with a major depression alone but that it was easier to return to a state of chronic or intermittent minor depression than to a self characterized by no depression at all (Keller & Shapiro, 1982). Among the 32 patients with double depression who recovered after 2 years of follow-up, 18 (56%) recovered from the major depression but not from the chronic minor depression and 13 (41%) recovered from both the major depression and the chronic depression.

In addition, patients with double depression had a higher rate of relapse and a faster cycle time for their major depressions over

**TABLE 4.2. Cumulative Probability (%) of Recovery of Patients with and without Double Depression**

| Number of weeks since entry into study | Recovery from MDD only | Recovery from MDD and dysthymic disorder |
|---|---|---|
| 4 | 18 | 3 |
| 8 | 33 | 6 |
| 12 | 49 | 8 |
| 26 | 69 | 20 |
| 52 | 83 | 29 |
| 78 | 93 | 38 |
| 104 | 97 | 43 |

*Note. n* (major depressive disorder only) = 236; *n* (double depression) = 80. MDD, major depressive disorder. From Keller, Lavori, Endicott, Coryell, & Klerman (1983). 

2 years. In the group of 133 patients who were observed for the entire 2-year follow-up period, 20 (63%) of the 32 patients with double depression completed at least one cycle of recovery and relapse within 2 years, compared with 33 (33%) of the 101 patients without double depression. There were at least two prospective recoveries in 50% of the patients with double depression compared with 27% of the patients with major depression alone. Thus, repeated episodes of major affective disorder were much more likely in patients who had double depression (Keller et al., 1983). From such data it is possible for the clinician to predict that a patient whose major depressive disorder is accompanied by a preexisting chronic minor depression is at very high risk for repetitive episodes of major affective disorder. Furthermore, the patient with double depression who arrives at a clinical state of recovery from the major depression is poised between two outcomes: a complete recovery (from the chronic minor depression) and a relapse into another major affective episode. The longer the patient remains chronically ill after recovering from the major depression, the greater the likelihood that relapse will preempt complete recovery (Keller, 1985; Keller et al., 1983).

Double depressives also differ from major depressives without underlying dysthymia in several other respects. Klein et al. (1988) compared 31 outpatients who met DSM-III criteria for both major depression and dysthymia to 50 outpatients who met DSM-III (American Psychiatric Association, 1980) criteria for episodic major depression in order to examine whether the groups differed on clinical, familial, and psychosocial characteristics. The subjects studied were outpatients from a community mental health center and a university-based clinic. Dated from the point when the full criteria were met, the duration of the current major depressive episode was found to be significantly shorter for patients with double depression than for the patients with episodic depression, suggesting that the severity of the depressions in the former group increased more rapidly or that the doubly depressed patients sought treatment more quickly than the patients with episodic depression. Further comparisons of patients with double depression versus episodic depression led to the following conclusions: (1) A significantly greater proportion of patients with double depression had a history of suicide attempts. (2) Patients with double depression reported a significantly poorer adolescent social adjustment and lower levels of social support. (3) Relatives of patients with double depression had significantly higher rates of bipolar II and nonbipolar depressive disorders. (4) Both parents of a significantly greater proportion of patients with double depression had an affective disorder. (5) Patients with double depression exhibited significantly higher mean levels of depression and poorer social and global functioning across a 6-month follow-up period (Klein et al., 1988).

## Dysthymic Disorder

Dysthymic disorder (or depressive neurosis) was defined in DSM-III as a persistently depressed mood or loss of pleasure that is present, with periods of normal mood lasting no longer than a few months, for at least 2 years (1 year for children) but is not of sufficient severity to warrant a diagnosis of major depression. During this episode, by definition, there are no delusions or hallucinations and the episode has a chronic course with no clear onset. DSM-III states that at least 3 of the following 13 symptoms must be present during the depressive episode: insomnia or hypersomnia; chronic tiredness or low energy level; feelings of inadequacy, loss of self-esteem, or self-deprecation; decreased effectiveness or productivity at school, work, or home; decreased attention, concentration, or ability to think clearly; social withdrawal; loss of interest in or enjoyment of pleasurable activities; irritability or excessive anger (in children, expressed toward parents or caretakers); inability to respond with apparent pleasure to praise or rewards; less active or talkative than usual or feelings of having slowed down; restlessness; pessimistic attitude toward the future; brooding about past events; self-pity, tearfulness or crying; and recurrent thoughts of death or suicide.

In DSM-III-R (American Psychiatric Association, 1987) dysthymia is similarly defined as the presence of a persistently depressed mood that lasts most of the day or is present more often than it is absent over a 2-year period. One major difference in the revised diagnosis is the choice of symptoms to be reported upon. In DSM-III 3 symptoms from a list of 13 symptoms were required for the diagnosis of dysthymia. For the DSM-III-R diagnosis of dysthymia, a patient must report at least two of the following six symptoms: poor appetite or overeating; insomnia or hypersomnia; low energy or fatigue; low self-esteem; poor concentration or difficulty in making decisions; and hopelessness. DSM-III-R also requires the specification of primary versus secondary type and early versus late onset. Early onset describes an onset before the age of 21; late onset describes an onset at the age of 21 or older. According to DSM-IV, dysthymic disorder may not be diagnosed if there has been an episode of major depression during the first 2 years of the disturbance (1 year for children and adolescents), in which case a diagnosis of chronic major depression or major depressive disorder, in partial remission, may be warranted. However, a diagnosis of dysthymic dosorder may be made, after a major depressive episode, if there are no significant signs or symptoms for 2 months (American Psychiatric Association, 1994).

Research has shown that a large majority of those from a clinical population who were diagnosed with dysthymia go on to develop a major depression (Keller & Lavori, 1984). For example, in a study conducted by Akiskal, King, Rosenthal, Robinson, and Scott-Strauss (1981), 90% of 137 outpatients originally diagnosed with dysthymic disorder were found to also suffer from major affective episodes. Moreover, in a prospective study of children it was found that over 70% of those originally diagnosed with dysthymia developed a major depression over a 5-year follow-up (Kovacs, Feinberg, Crouse-Novak, Paulauskas, & Finkelstein, 1984).

The epidemiology of dysthymia (called chronic depression in the earlier research) has been studied by various groups, including Weissman, Leaf, Bruce, and Florio (1988), Karno et al. (1987), Myers et al. (1984), and Robins et al. (1984). Dysthymia has been found to be common in these studies of community samples, with a prevalence of 2.7% to 4.3%.

## Duration

Several studies have examined the duration of a dysthymic episode. In children the average length of a dysthymic episode is significantly longer than a major depression, with 3 years being the average length for dysthymia and 32 weeks for a major depressive episode (Kovacs et al., 1984). The duration can range from 2 to 20 years in studies of adult dysthymics, with a median duration of approximately 5 years (Keller & Shapiro, 1982; Rounsaville, Shokomskas, & Prusoff, 1980). This long duration is partly expected on the basis of the definitions of the criteria.

## Recovery

It is important to diagnose both major depression and dysthymia in order to assess outcome (Keller & Shapiro, 1982). As discussed earlier, a 2-year follow-up study by Keller and Lavori (1984) found that 97% of a group of double depressives had recovered from their major depressive disorder, but only 39% had recovered from the underlying acute and chronic phases of dysthymia. In other words, after 2 years, 61% of the patients with double depression had not recovered from the underlying dysthymic disorder (Keller et al., 1983). In another 2-year naturalistic follow-up study, Barrett (1984) found that 63% of the subjects claimed to experience no improvement, with some stating that they were suffering from a more severe illness.

## Relapse/Recurrence

Keller et al. (1983) studied a group of 66 patients who were originally diagnosed with double depression and who had recovered from their major depression. These patients were studied at 6-month intervals over a 1-year period to determine the rate of relapse. Overall, in that year 25 (38%) of the patients recovered from the chronic minor depression, 24 (36%) had relapsed into a RDC major affective disorder, and 17 (26%) remained in a state of chronic minor depression. In the first 6 months of the year, 20 patients (30%) recovered from their chronic minor depression, 12 (18%) relapsed into a major affective disorder, and 34 (52%) remained in a chronic depression. Of the 34 patients remaining in a chronic minor depression at the second 6-month interval, 5 (15%) recovered from their chronic minor depression and 12 (35%) relapsed into a major affective disorder. This study indicates that over a 1-year period, dysthymic patients have an increased chance of relapse into a major affective episode and a decreased chance of recovery from a chronic minor depression.

Distinctions between chronic major depression and dysthymia are controversial but are seemingly becoming more imperative in order to afford the patient the best chance of recovery. Some research supports the belief that it would be best to differentiate dysthymia from major depression in terms of severity and chronicity differences rather than qualitative differences. The most typical course would consist of an insidious onset of symptoms at an early age followed by a fluctuating or progressive course that will often meet current diagnostic criteria for major depression. This may represent a more severe and malevolent form of typical recurrent unipolar affective disorder than the episodic type, as suggested by the reports of increased family rates of affective illness and poor outcome. Some of these cases, however, seem highly responsive to treatment with antidepressant medication. The differences are quantitative, being based on severity and chronicity, and not qualitative. The general feeling among most researchers is that whenever dysthymia and major depression coexist, regardless of which came first, a unitary phenomenon is occurring (Keller & Russell, in press).

## DSM-IV Mood Disorders Field Trial

Due to the need for further investigation regarding the relationship between major depression and dysthymia and in preparation for the fourth edition of the DSM, a DSM-IV Field Trial for Dysthymia, Major Depression, Minor Depression, and Depressive Personality was conducted. Five sites were involved in the field trial: Butler Hospital, Brown University; Virginia Commonwealth University; the Payne Whitney Clinic, Cornell University; the State

University of New York at Stony Brook; and the University of Texas Medical Branch at Galveston. Approximately 100 subjects at each site (517 total) were recruited from clinical inpatient and outpatient settings and from community sources (Keller et al., in press).

The field trial attempted to address a number of concerns regarding the DSM-III-R definition of dysthymia, including the following: (1) the defining symptoms did not include many of those symptoms thought to be most characteristic of the disorder, (2) the threshold-defining criterion for case inclusion (i.e., number of symptoms required) was not empirically derived, and (3) the symptoms included in the criteria for major depression and dysthymia overlapped. The field trial also explored the need for additional categories for milder forms of mood disorder (e.g., minor and recurrent brief depression), examined the reliability of the methods used to measure personality disorder and the validity of the entity as distinct from dysthymia, and developed a nosology of mood disorders based on longitudinal course (Keller et al., in press). This chapter summarizes the data on the last issue, the development of a set of longitudinal course modifiers to be used in diagnosing depressive disorders.

## Course Modifiers for Major Depressive Disorder

Since the early 1980s, naturalistic follow-up and long-term treatment studies have challenged the traditional conception of the course of depression as an episodic and remitting illness. The traditional approach to classifying depression has emphasized cross-sectional symptomatology. Owing to recent studies suggesting that course-based characteristics such as recurrence, presence of prior dysthymia, duration of the index episode, and age of onset seem to have greater prognostic and treatment validity (Zimmerman & Spitzer, 1989), a course-based classification system was designed to supplement the traditional method of classification.

This system is based on three key considerations of the course of major depression: whether antecedent dysthymia is present or absent; whether episodes are single or recurrent; and whether, in the case of major depressions, there was full recovery between the two most recent episodes. These three factors can be combined to yield seven possible course types: (1) single episode with antecedent dysthymia; (2) single episode without antecedent dysthymia;

(3) recurrent with antecedent dysthymia and full interepisode recovery; (4) recurrent with antecedent dysthymia and without full interepisode recovery; (5) recurrent without antecedent dysthymia and with full interepisode recovery; (6) recurrent without antecedent dysthymia and without full interepisode recovery; and (7) unspecified, a residual category of cases that cannot be otherwise classified (Keller et al., in press).

One of the major goals of the DSM-IV Field Trial for Dysthymia, Major Depression, Minor Depression, and Depressive Personality was to examine the reliability and utility of this proposed longitudinal course-based nosology of major depression. In the field trial study, 432 subjects were diagnosed as having a current major depression on the Structured Clinical Interview for DSM-III-R (SCID). Using the proposed course modifiers, 384 (89%) of these subjects had a course modifier coded (see Table 4.3).

It was found that the relative frequencies of the specific course patterns were consistent with what has been reported in the literature and that few subjects failed to be assigned to a specific course type. For the most part, the proportions of subjects with each course pattern were relatively similar for most sites. The course modifiers generally exhibited acceptable levels, both within and across sites, of interrater reliability, and while there was some

**TABLE 4.3. Frequency of Occurrence of Course Modifier Types in 384 Depressives from the DSM-IV Mood Disorders Field Trial Investigation**

| Course type | *n* | % |
|---|---|---|
| Single episode with antecedent dysthymia | 33 | 8.6 |
| Single episode without antecedent dysthymia | 87 | 22.7 |
| Recurrent with antecedent dysthymia and with full recovery | 16 | 4.2 |
| Recurrent with antecedent dysthymia and without full recovery | 97 | 25.3 |
| Recurrent without antecedent dysthymia and with full recovery | 77 | 20.1 |
| Recurrent without antecedent dysthymia and without full recovery | 69 | 17.9 |
| Unspecified | 5 | 1.3 |

*Note.* From Keller (1994). Copyright 1994 by Munksgaard International Publishers, Ltd. Reprinted by permission.

variability in the reliability of the specific course types, none of the modifiers produced consistently poor kappas across analyses.

The American Psychiatric Association Task Force accepted the recommendation from the DSM-IV field trial investigators that course modifier graphs be included in the mood disorders section of DSM-IV to help clinicians differentially subtype the courses of dysthymic disorder and major depressive disorder (see Figure 4.1). This differential subtyping should be undertaken by carefully reviewing the duration and severity of the clinical course, beginning with the initial index episode of depression. Clinicians may find it helpful to graph the course of the disorder with the assistance of the patient (Keller et al., in press).

## Conclusion

Depression is a chronic, recurrent, insidious illness that can result in serious mental and physical health problems if it goes undiagnosed or undertreated. Epidemiologic Catchment Area data estimate an 8% lifetime prevalence rate in the general population, demonstrating that depression is one of the most common psychiatric disorders, yet the illness remains largely undetected by physi-

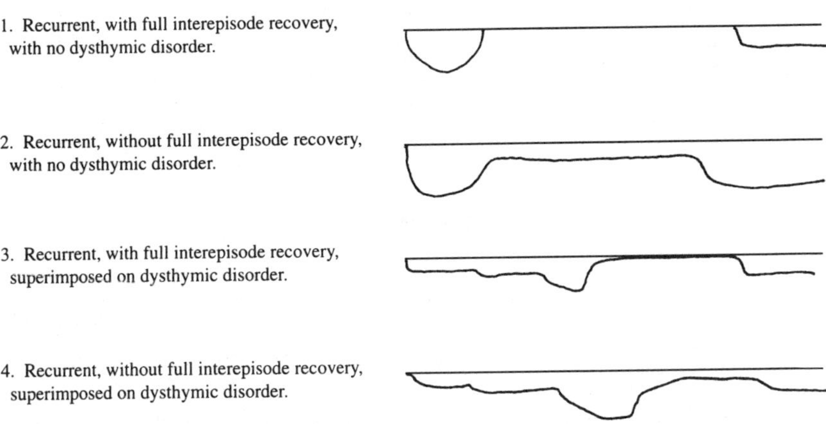


**FIGURE 4.1.** Longitudinal course modifiers for DSM-IV major depression. From American Psychiatric Association (1994). Copyright 1994 by the American Psychiatric Association. Reprinted by permission.

cians. Recent studies have shown that 50% of the people who suffer from depressive symptoms seek help from a nonpsychiatric medical clinician rather than a psychiatrist. Moreover, a significant percentage of primary care physicians fail to diagnose depression in their patients (Perez-Stable, Miranda, Munoz, & Ying, 1990). This is of great concern since some experts estimate that as many as 95% of people with mental and emotional disorders are treated by a general practitioner (Wilkinson, 1989). One explanation for the fact that patients suffering from depression seek out a nonpsychiatric medical clinician is that they are experiencing poor physical functioning. In fact, studies have shown that current health, role functioning, and social functioning are all worse in patients with depressive symptoms than in those with such chronic illnesses as hypertension, diabetes, arthritis, gastrointestinal disorders, and lung disorders (Wells et al., 1989).

As a medical disorder, depressive illness is comparable to diabetes or hypertension in that a meaningful proportion of patients have a chronic or recurrent course, with substantial impairment in functioning, morbidity, and mortality. Long-term maintenance treatment, as with any chronic disease, is critical to recovery and the avoidance of recurrence. Immediate recognition of this illness and intervention are essential in effecting a rapid recovery and in preventing further acute affective episodes. In the past several years new classes of antidepressant medications that are highly effective and have less harmful side effects have become available. Unfortunately, chronic depression remains undertreated, as do acute episodes of major depression (Keller, 1990).

## References

Akiskal, H. S., King, D., Rosenthal, T. L., Robinson, D., & Scott-Strauss, A. (1981). Chronic depression: Part I. Clinical and familial characteristics in 137 probands. *Journal of Affective Disorders*, *3*, 297–315.

American Psychiatric Association. (1980). *Diagnostic and statistical manual of mental disorders* (3rd ed.). Washington, DC: Author.

American Psychiatric Association. (1987). *Diagnostic and statistical manual of mental disorders* (3rd ed., rev.). Washington, DC: Author.

American Psychiatric Association. (1994). *Diagnostic and statistical manual of mental disorders* (4th ed.). Washington, DC: Author.

Barrett, J. (1984). Naturalistic change over two years in neurotic depressive disorders (RDC categories). *Comprehensive Psychiatry, 25*(4), 404–418.

Karno, M., Hough, R. L., Burnam, A. M., Escobar, J. I., Timbers, D. M., Santana, F., & Boyd, J. H. (1987). Lifetime psychiatric disorders among Mexican-Americans and non-Hispanic whites in Los Angeles. *Archives of General Psychiatry, 44*, 695–701.

Keller, M. B. (1985). Chronic and recurrent affective disorders: Incidence, course, and influencing factors. In D. Kemali & G. Racagni (Eds.), *Chronic treatments in neuropsychiatry* (pp. 111–119). New York: Raven Press.

Keller, M. B. (1990). Depression: Underrecognition and undertreatment by psychiatrists and other health care professionals. *Archives of Internal Medicine, 150*, 946–948.

Keller, M. B. (1994). Course, outcome and impact on the community. *Acta Psychiatrica Scandinavica, 89* (Suppl. 383), 24–34.

Keller, M. B., Hirschfeld, R. M. A., Klein, D. N., Kocsis, J. H. McCullough, J. P., Miller, I., First, M., Holzer, C. P., Keitner, G. I., Marin, D. B., & Shea, M. T. (in press). DSM-IV Mood Disorders Field Trial investigation results. *American Journal of Psychiatry.*

Keller, M. B., & Lavori, P. W. (1984). Double depression, major depression and dysthymia: Distinct entities or different phases of a single disorder? *Psychopharmacology Bulletin, 20*, 399–402.

Keller, M. B., Lavori, P. W., Endicott, J., Coryell, W., & Klerman, G. L. (1983). "Double depression": A two-year follow-up. *American Journal of Psychiatry, 140*, 689–694.

Keller, M. B., Lavori, P. W., Mueller, T. I., Endicott, J., Coryell, W., Hirschfeld, R. M. A., & Shea, T. (1992). Time to recovery, chronicity, and levels of psychopathology in major depression. *Archives of General Psychiatry, 49*, 809–816.

Keller, M. B., & Russell, C. W. (in press). Dysthymia. In T. Widiger, A. Frances, & H. Pincus (Eds.), *DSM-IV sourcebook*. Washington, DC: American Psychiatric Association Press.

Keller, M. B., & Shapiro, R. W. (1982). "Double depression": Superimposition of acute depressive episodes on chronic depressive disorders. *American Journal of Psychiatry, 139*(4), 438–442.

Klein, D., Taylor, E., Harding, K., & Dickstein, S. (1988). Double depression and episodic major depression: Demographic, clinical, familial, personality and socio-environmental characteristics and short-term outcome. *American Journal of Psychiatry, 145*, 10.

Kovacs, M., Feinberg, T. L., Crouse-Novak, M., Paulauskas, S. L., & Finkelstein, R. (1984). Depressive disorders in childhood: I. A longitudinal prospective study of characteristics and recovery. *Archives of General Psychiatry, 41,* 229–237.

Myers, J. M., Weissman, M. M., Tischeler, G. L., Holzer, C. E. Leaf, P. J., Orvaschel, H., Antony, J. V., Boyd, J. H., Burke, J. D., Kramer, M., & Stolzman, R. (1984). Six-month prevalence of psychiatric disorders in three communities, 1980–1982. *Archives of General Psychiatry, 41,* 959–967.

Perez-Stable, E. J., Miranda, J., Munoz, R. F., & Ying, Y.-W. (1990). Depression in medical outpatients: Underrecognition and misdiagnosis. *Archives of Internal Medicine, 150,* 1083–1088.

Regier, D. A., Boyd, J. H., Burke, J. D., Rae, D. S., Kramer, M., Robins, L. N., George, L. K., Karno, M., & Locke, B. Z. (1988). One-month prevalence of mental disorders in the United States: Based on five Epidemiologic Catchment Area sites. *Archives of General Psychiatry, 45,* 977–986.

Robins, L. N., Helzer, J. E., Weissman, M. M., Orvaschel, H., Gruenberg, E., Burke, J. D., & Regier, D. A. (1984). Lifetime prevalence of specific psychiatric disorders in three sites. *Archives of General Psychiatry, 41,* 949–958.

Rounsaville, B. J., Shokomskas, D., & Prusoff, B. A. (1980). Chronic mood disorders in depressed outpatients: Diagnosis and response to pharmacotherapy. *Journal of Affective Disorders, 2,* 72–88.

Weissman, M. M., Leaf, P. J., Bruce, M. L., & Florio, L. (1988). The epidemiology of dysthymia in five communities: Rates, risks, comorbidity and treatment. *American Journal of Psychiatry, 145,* 815–819.

Wells, K. B., Stewart, A., Hays, R. D., Burnam, M. A., Rogers, W., Daniels, M., Berry, S., Greenfield, S., & Ware, J. (1989). The functioning and well-being of depressed patients: Results from the medical outcomes study. *Journal of the American Medical Association, 262,* 914–919.

Wilkinson, G. (1989). Research report: The General Practice Research Unit at the Institute of Psychiatry. *Psychological Medicine, 19,* 789–790.

Zimmerman, M., & Spitzer, R. (1989). Melancholia: From DSM-III to DSM-III-R. *American Journal of Psychiatry, 146*(1), 20–28.

CHAPTER FIVE

# Assessment of Symptoms and Change in Dysthymic Disorder

BARBARA J. MASON
JAMES H. KOCSIS
ANDREW C. LEON
SETH THOMPSON
ALLEN J. FRANCES
ROBERT O. MORGAN
MICHAEL K. PARIDES

Data from dysthymic disorder treatment trials reviewed in Chapters 8 and 9 of this volume suggest that interventions initially developed for treating episodic major depressions may be modified to treat the chronic symptomatology of dysthymic disorder. However, controlled clinical trials require a valid measure of baseline severity and clinical change as well as criteria for response. Assessment of clinical response in dysthymic disorder may have been limited by the structure and format of existing rating instruments (Spitzer & Williams, 1985). For example, the Hamilton Rating Scale for Depression (HRSD) and the Beck Depression Inventory (BDI) have generally served as the standard instruments for measurement of depressive severity in clinical trials of major depressive disorder (Beck, Ward, Mendelson, Mock, & Erbaugh, 1961; Hamilton,

1960). The HRSD is administered by a trained interviewer; the BDI is commonly used as a self-report instrument.

The HRSD was developed to assess endogenously depressed inpatients and is heavily weighted toward neurovegetative symptoms associated with response to somatic therapies in major depression. However, patients with dysthymic disorder frequently lack typical neurovegetative symptoms but report a high prevalence of cognitive and behavioral symptoms, such as poor self-esteem and social withdrawal (Keller et al., in press; Kocsis & Frances, 1987). Moreover, the HRSD yields a restricted range of possible scores with which to assess change in dysthymic patients. Specifically, 10 items of the 24-item version of the HRSD have only three possible severity ratings: 0, 1, or 2. The remaining items are rated on a 5-point scale ranging from 0 to 4. Many of the severity ratings of 3 or 4 require psychosis or a severity level not otherwise found in an outpatient dysthymic sample. Hence, the HRSD yields a restricted range of possible scores with which to assess baseline severity and change in dysthymic patients. Furthermore, since the HRSD and the BDI were developed to measure episodic rather than chronic states of depression, items are cued to comparisons with recent normal premorbid periods (Beck et al., 1961). On the basis of these considerations we sought to develop appropriate symptom-based rating scales, in both interviewer and self-rated versions, to measure symptom intensity, clinical change, and response to treatment in chronic depression of mild to moderate severity.

A rating scale for dysthymic disorder was felt to require the following: (1) the capacity to assess the milder symptomatology of chronically depressed outpatients, (2) the capacity to assess characteristic symptomatology (i.e., with a weighting toward cognitive and behavioral symptoms rather than neurovegetative symptoms), and (3) anchor points relating to current and recent frequency and severity of symptoms rather than to normal premorbid periods. It was hypothesized that scales developed specifically to rate severity and measure change in dysthymia would be more sensitive to the symptomatology characteristic of dysthymic patients and to change in response to treatment of dysthymia than are traditional rating scales of major depression such as the HRSD and BDI.

# Development of the Cornell Dysthymia Rating Scale

## Subjects and Method

The first step in generating an interviewer-administered rating scale for dysthymia was to systematically and comprehensively identify those symptoms most descriptive of dysthymic disorder. A 19-item 5-point scale was constructed to assess symptoms potentially descriptive of dysthymia that were not adequately assessed by the 24-item HRSD. These items were derived from the DSM-III (American Psychiatric Association, 1980) list of associated symptoms for dysthymic disorder and from the Research Diagnostic Criteria (RDC) list of associated symptoms for minor depression (Spitzer, Endicott, & Robins, 1978). Altogether, the HRSD and the DSM-III/RDC symptom list comprised 43 items.

Ratings were made by research psychiatrists or psychologists on these 43 items in 55 subjects with primary DSM-III dysthymic disorder who were psychiatric outpatients participating in a clinical trial of imipramine (IMI) for the treatment of chronic depression (Kocsis et al., 1988). Ratings were made prior to treatment in 17 men and 38 women (mean age = 38.6 years, *SD* = 12.8; mean duration of reported depression = 22.6 years, *SD* = 17.2). Frequency distributions were computed for all items studied. Items were considered to be frequently endorsed if rated at a severity rating of mild or greater by at least 67% of the sample. In order to identify overlapping DSM-III/RDC dysthymia symptoms and HRSD items, the correlations between these sets were computed. Similarly worded items that were correlated .5 or higher were consolidated into a single item in order to reduce redundancy.

## Results

Twelve items from the DSM-III/RDC symptom list were rated as present by at least two-thirds of the sample. These items included dysphoria, disturbed sleep, tiredness, feelings of inadequacy, decreased effectiveness, decreased concentration, social withdrawal, loss of interest, irritability, pessimism, worry, and indecisiveness. Twelve HRSD items also met these criteria and included depressed mood, guilt, suicidal ideation, decreased activity, psychic anxiety, somatic anxiety, somatic symptoms, sexual symptoms, diurnal variation, hopelessness, helplessness, and feelings of worthlessness. Infrequently endorsed items from the DSM-III/RDC symptom list included unresponsiveness to praise, uncommunicativeness, tearfulness, recurrent suicidal ideation, self-pity, hypersomnia, and hyperphagia. Infrequently endorsed HRSD items included all three insomnia items (early, middle, and late), psychomotor retardation and agitation, gastrointestinal symptoms, hypochondriasis, weight loss, lack of insight, depersonalization, paranoia, and obsessiveness.

Dysphoria, feelings of inadequacy, pessimism, and decreased effectiveness on the DSM III/RDC symptom list correlated at a level of .5 or greater with depressed mood, feelings of worthlessness, feelings of helplessness, and decreased work and activities on the HRSD, respectively. These similarly worded items were consolidated into single items. In this manner the final Cornell Dysthymia Rating Scale (CDRS) was developed to include 20 items.

A 5-point scale (ranging from 0 to 4) was developed for all items on the CDRS. Statements depicting five gradations of frequency or severity relevant to dysthymia were included for each item, using a format similar to the Schedule for Affective Disorders and Schizophrenia (Endicott & Spitzer, 1979). In this format each item can be rated from 0 (symptom absent) to 4 (severe). For all items, a higher score corresponds to greater symptom severity. Examples of the format used in the final CDRS are presented in Figure 5.1. Raters are instructed to assess severity of symptoms from the 2-week period prior to treatment in order to establish baseline measures and then for each subsequent rating interval.

## A Comparison of Dysthymia Severity Ratings with the CDRS and Existing Rating Instruments

### Subjects and Method

The sample of patients used in comparison studies of the CDRS and existing rating instruments consisted of 108 patients (39 males and 69 females with a mean age of 37 years, *SD* = 11) with dysthymia who had participated either in a double-blind clinical trial of IMI ($n = 20$)

|  |  |
|---|---|
| **1. DEPRESSED MOOD**<br>Subjective feelings of depression based on verbal complaints of feeling depressed, sad, blue, gloomy, down in the dumps, empty, "don't care." Do not include such ideational aspects as discouragement, pessimism, and feelings of worthlessness or suicide attempts (all of which are to be rated separately). | ☐ Not at all<br>☐ Slight (e.g., only occasionally feels "sad" or down)<br>☐ Mild (e.g., often feels somewhat "depressed," blue, or downhearted<br>☐ Moderate (e.g., most of the time feels depressed)<br>☐ Severe (e.g., most of the time feels "very depressed" or "miserable") |
| **2. LACK OF INTEREST OR PLEASURE:**<br>Pervasive lack of interest in work, family, friends, sex, hobbies, and other leisure-time activities. Severity is determined by the number of important activities in which the subject has less interest or pleasure compared to nonpatients. | ☐ All activities as interesting or pleasurable<br>☐ 1 or 2 activities less interesting or pleasurable<br>☐ Several activities less interesting or pleasurable<br>☐ Most activities less interesting or pleasurable with one or two exceptions<br>☐ Total absence of pleasure in almost all activities |
| **3. PESSIMISM:**<br>Discouragement, pessimism, and hopelessness | ☐ Not at all discouraged about the future<br>☐ Slight (e.g., occasional feelings of mild discouragement about the future)<br>☐ Mild (e.g., often somewhat discouraged but can usually be talked into feeling hopeful)<br>☐ Moderate (e.g., often feels quite pessimistic about the future and can only sometimes be talked into feeling hopeful)<br>☐ Severe (e.g., pervasive feelings of intense pessimism or hopelessness) |

**FIGURE 5.1.** Examples of three CDRS items.

versus placebo ($n = 20$) or in the open label phase of a desipramine (DMI) maintenance study ($n = 68$). Subjects met DSM-III criteria for dysthymic disorder, based on a Structured Clinical Interview for DSM-III (SCID), and were excluded if they had an organic, psychotic, or substance use disorder or a significant medical disorder that contraindicated the use of tricyclic antidepressants (Spitzer & Williams, 1985). Since we wished to develop a rating instrument applicable across the range of severity of dysthymia, patients were included whether or not they met current or past criteria for major depression. Baseline ratings were obtained with the CDRS, HRSD, and Global Assessment Scale (GAS) (Endicott, Spitzer, Fleiss, & Cohen, 1976).

The GAS is a global psychopathology scale with higher scores indicating better function. A subsample of 50 subjects (33 subjects from the IMI study and 17 from the DMI study) also completed the 21-item self-rated BDI.

## Results

### Distribution of Severity Ratings

Distributional statistics were compared for baseline severity ratings on the CDRS and HRSD items and total scale scores. Because the scaling of the CDRS items was designed to allow raters to differentiate across a milder range of depressive symptomatology, it was hypothesized that the CDRS would yield a broader range of scores and more endorsed items than the HRSD. This hypothesis was supported: A full range of possible severity ratings (0 to 4) on the CDRS was endorsed on all items. Conversely, a full range of possible severity scores was found on only 3 of the 14 HRSD items (which have a range of 5 points). Similarly, the mean severity rating was greater than 1.0 on only 10 of the 24 HRSD items. CDRS total scores at baseline ranged from 14 to 63 with a mean of 40.1 and a standard deviation of 10.3. The baseline HRSD total scores ranged from 7 to 41, with a mean of 21.3 and a standard deviation of 7.1. A graphic depiction of mean severity ratings on similar CDRS and HRSD items is presented in Figure 5.2. A comparison of CDRS, HRSD, and BDI mean total scores at baseline and at Week 6 and the change in scores (baseline minus Week 6) is depicted in Figure 5.3. Week 6 total CDRS and HRSD scores showed similar average rates of change from baseline: 38% and 42%, respectively. However, as at baseline, the CDRS showed a broader range of scores (0 to 59) than the HRSD (0 to 35) at Week 6. The BDI showed a smaller rate of change than the CDRS or HRSD, with the mean total score changing only 26.9% from baseline.

### Convergent Validity

Convergent validity for the CDRS was assessed by examining the degree of association of scores from the CDRS with data from three frequently used measures of depression and global psychopathology:

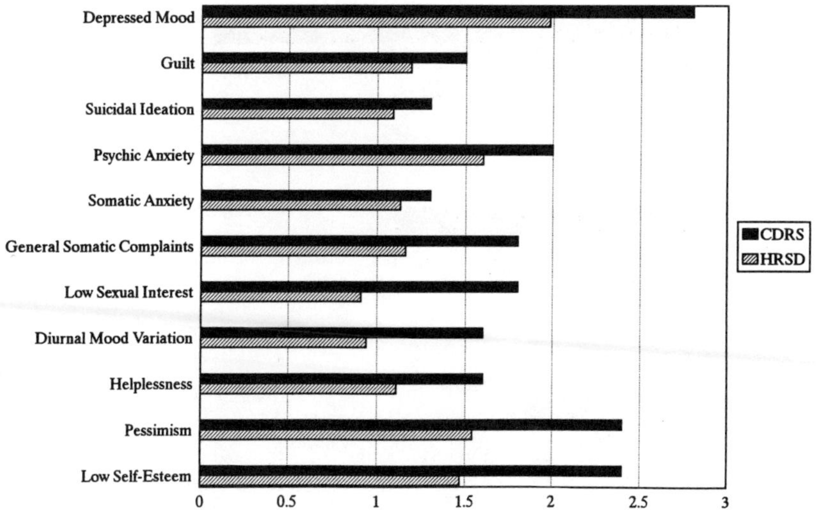


**FIGURE 5.2.** Comparison of mean baseline severity ratings on corresponding items from the CDRS and HRSD. Higher scores indicate greater symptom severity. $n$ = 108.

the HRSD, the BDI, and the GAS. CDRS total scores were significantly correlated (all $p$ values $< .001$ except where indicated) with HRSD scores at baseline ($r = .65$), Week 6 ($r = .83$), and in terms of change scores (baseline minus Week 6 ratings; $r = .80$). Similarly, the CDRS correlated significantly with the BDI at baseline ($r = .44$, $p = .004$), Week 6 ($r = .62$), and in terms of change scores ($r = .65$). In addition, the CDRS showed the expected significant inverse correlations with the GAS (baseline, $r = -.53$; Week 6, $r = -.74$; change, $r = -.71$). These relationships between the CDRS and other depression and functional measures suggest good convergent validity. The scores from the CDRS did not correlate significantly with demographic characteristics of the sample.

## The CDRS as a Measure of Response to Treatment

The milder, more chronic symptoms of dysthymia, relative to major depressive disorder, require that a strict definition of re-

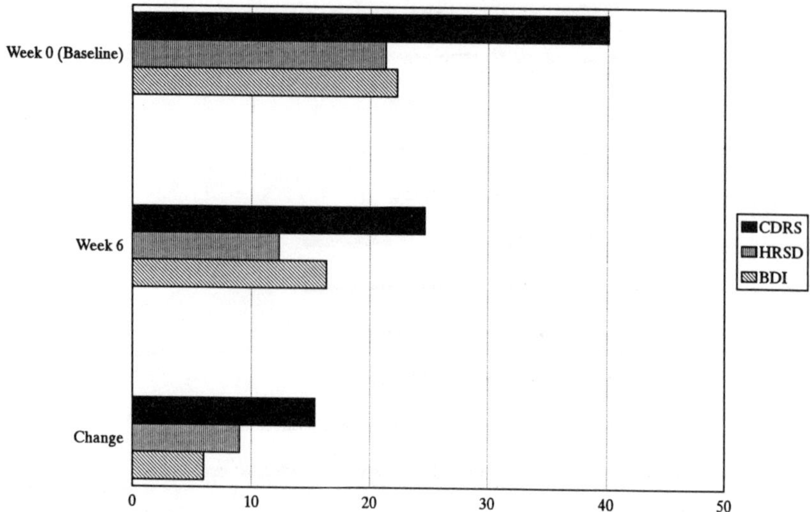


**FIGURE 5.3.** Mean total scores at Week 0 and at Week 6 and change scores for the CDRS, HRSD, and BDI.

sponse be employed in dysthymia treatment trials, namely, minimal to absent symptoms of depression with the patient no longer meeting syndromal criteria for dysthymia. Given a minimum threshold for entry into a treatment trial, this strict definition of response should minimize the placebo response rate and distinguish effective treatments. Consequently, responders for these analyses were defined as having Week 6 HRSD total scores less than 7 and at least a 10-point increase in GAS score from baseline. Nonresponders were those patients not meeting these criteria.

## Subjects and Method

Subjects described earlier in the CDRS comparison studies section were evaluated for response following completion of 6 weeks of treatment. Baseline and Week 6 scores were compared from the 20-item CDRS and the 24-item HRSD. Point biserial correlations were computed between change scores and responder status. Receiver Operating Characteristic (ROC) curves were used to determine optimal CDRS scores for identifying response or nonresponse to treatment using the aforementioned definition (Hsiao, Bartko, & Potter, 1989). ROC curves are a visual representation of the comparative increases in true positive versus false positive diagnoses as a diagnostic cutoff point is moved from one end of the scale score continuum to the other. Thus, the ROC curve provides information about both the sensitivity (the true positive rate) and the specificity (the true negative rate) of a diagnostic measure.

## Results

After 6 weeks of drug treatment, there were significant reductions from baseline in CDRS and HRSD total scores. The CDRS change score had a slightly stronger correlation with responder/nonresponder status ($r$ = .54) than the HRSD did ($r$ = .48). This is intriguing given that the HRSD was used as a partial determinant of response status and the CDRS was not.

Inspection of the area under the ROC curve of the CDRS revealed that a cutoff score of 20 correctly identified 94.3% of treatment responders (true positives) and incorrectly identified 16.4% of nonresponders as responders (false positives). Higher cutoff scores increased the rate of both true and false positives, and conversely, lower cutoff scores decreased the rate of both true and false positives.

## Development of the Cornell Dysthymia Rating Scale–Self-Report

It was felt that a valid self-report instrument for measuring baseline severity and change in dysthymic symptoms required the following: (1) clarity, so that self-administration would be unambiguous; (2) brevity; (3) items that address all symptoms characteristic of dysthymia; and (4) standardized anchor points that quantify symptom severity so that individual patient scores, research data sets, and other quantitative data can be meaningfully compared and so that improvement in response to treatment can be objectively demonstrated. Furthermore, a self-report instrument was felt to require a design that permitted easy identification of any items that the patient may have omitted to answer and identification of any response bias, for example, consistently endorsing a mid-range of severity across items.

## Subjects and Method

The Zung Depression Scale uses a grid format with four columns to depict item severity (Zung, 1965). A modification of this format was applied to the Cornell Dysthymia Rating Scale–Self-Report (CDRS-SR) so that the researcher or clinician who retrieves the scale from the patient can quickly scan the grid to identify any omitted items or an invalid response set. Items of the CDRS-SR are listed vertically in the grid and are rated across four columns with the following headings: (1) None or a little of the time, (2) Some of the time, (3) Good part of the time, and (4) Most or all of the time. Some items are worded in a positive fashion (e.g., "I enjoy receiving praise or compliments") while other items are negatively worded (e.g., "I have trouble sleeping at night"). Thus, for example, if the extreme left columns are consistently checked, further inquiry should be initiated to determine if a response set to use the "none or a little of the time" rating has resulted in an invalid self-assessment. (An even number of columns eliminates the possibility of a middle-column response set.) A key for scoring the CDRS-SR is presented in Table 5.1, which illustrates how such an invalid response set can be easily determined by a quick visual scan.

Inclusion of symptoms in the CDRS-SR was empirically determined and not based on theory pertaining to etiology or underlying causes of dysthymia. A 29-item pilot version of the CDRS-SR was developed on the basis of the empirically determined items of the CDRS and on the characteristic attitudes and symptoms of dysthymic patients recorded by the senior author of this chapter in the course of her treatment of dysthymic patients (Mason, Markowitz, & Klerman, 1993). The last 62 patients who participated in the psychometric studies of the CDRS also rated themselves with this pilot version of the CDRS-SR prior to beginning treatment for dysthymia.

Frequency distributions were computed for each item of the pilot version of the CDRS-SR. For all items, a score of 1 indicated minimal or absent symptoms and higher ratings indicated greater

**TABLE 5.1. Key for Scoring the Cornell Dysthymia Rating Scale–Self-Report (CDRS-SR)**

| | Scale item | None or a little of the time | Some of the time | Good part of the time | Most or all of the time |
|---|---|---|---|---|---|
| 1. | I feel sad, blue, down in the dumps, low. | 1 | 2 | 3 | 4 |
| 2. | I have trouble sleeping at night. | 1 | 2 | 3 | 4 |
| 3. | My physical energy is low. I feel tired or slowed down for no reason and am less active or talkative than I should be. | 1 | 2 | 3 | 4 |
| 4. | I feel inadequate, inferior, worthless, *no good.* | 1 | 2 | 3 | 4 |
| 5. | I am productive and effective in my job/school/home. | 4 | 3 | 2 | 1 |
| 6. | I have difficulty concentrating or remembering things. | 1 | 2 | 3 | 4 |
| 7. | I socialize as much as I would like to. | 4 | 3 | 2 | 1 |
| 8. | I am able to enjoy and to take pleasure in things. | 4 | 3 | 2 | 1 |
| 9. | I am more irritable or angry than I should be. | 1 | 2 | 3 | 4 |
| 10. | I enjoy receiving praise or compliments. | 4 | 3 | 2 | 1 |
| 11. | I feel hopeless, doubtful that things will improve. | 1 | 2 | 3 | 4 |
| 12. | I cry or feel tearful. | 1 | 2 | 3 | 4 |
| 13. | I think of dying or wish I was dead. | 1 | 2 | 3 | 4 |
| 14. | I feel sorry for myself. | 1 | 2 | 3 | 4 |
| 15. | I worry too much about things. | 1 | 2 | 3 | 4 |
| 16. | It is easy for me to make decisions. | 4 | 3 | 2 | 1 |
| 17. | I am as interested in sex as most people my age are. | 4 | 3 | 2 | 1 |
| 18. | I feel guilty. | 1 | 2 | 3 | 4 |
| 19. | I have trouble saying no to people and asserting myself. | 1 | 2 | 3 | 4 |
| 20. | I have trouble making and keeping close adult relationships. | 1 | 2 | 3 | 4 |
| 21. | It is easy for me to adjust to new circumstances. | 4 | 3 | 2 | 1 |
| 22. | I can handle criticism or rejection without getting upset. | 4 | 3 | 2 | 1 |
| 23. | I expect that people will be trustworthy and will treat me in a way that I will be comfortable with. | 4 | 3 | 2 | 1 |
| 24. | I can be cheered up easily. | 4 | 3 | 2 | 1 |
| 25. | It is easy for me to get started once I have decided to do something. | 4 | 3 | 2 | 1 |
| 26. | My appetite is poor, or I tend to overeat. | 1 | 2 | 3 | |
| 27. | My arms and legs feel heavy or weighted down. | 1 | 2 | 3 | 4 |

symptom severity. Thus, as with the CDRS, items were considered frequently endorsed if rated at a severity level of 2 or greater by at least 67% of the sample. Overlapping items were identified by generating a correlation matrix of all items. Items that had similar content and that correlated .5 or higher were consolidated into a single item in order to reduce redundancy.

## Results

Three items did not meet criteria for being frequently endorsed and were eliminated from the final version of the CDRS-SR: psychomotor agitation ("I feel restless, fidgety, like I can't sit still"), hypersomnia ("I am sleeping too much or spending too much time in bed"), and hyperphagia ("My appetite is too great; I crave foods"). However, given that DSM-IV (American Psychiatric Association, 1994) criteria for dysthymic disorder include a feature pertaining to poor appetite or overeating, the following item was included in the final version of the CDRS-SR: "My appetite is poor, or I tend to overeat."

Two items pertaining to low energy ("My physical energy is low, and I feel tired for no reason") and feeling slowed down ("I feel slowed down and am less active or talkative that I should be") were significantly correlated ($r = .53, p < .001$) and were sufficiently similar in content to be consolidated into one item in order to reduce redundancy on the scale: "My physical energy is low. I feel tired or slowed down for no reason and am less active or talkative than I should be." An item pertaining to feelings of leaden paralysis was not included in the pilot version of the CDRS-SR, but since one is included in the DSM-IV atypical features specifier that can be applied to dysthymic disorder, the following item was added to the final version of the CDRS-SR: "My arms and legs feel heavy or weighted down."

Six additional pairs of items had correlations greater than .5 but did not have overlapping content requiring consolidation into a single item: Dysphoric mood was associated with low energy ($r = .58, p < .001$) and inactivity ($r = .53, p < .001$). Poor self-esteem correlated with hopelessness ($r = .61, p < .001$). Persons who indicated that they socialized less than they would like to also indicated that they had less interest in sex relative to most people their age ($r = .52, p < .001$).

Persons who felt that they worried too much also tended to feel greater guilt ($r = .58$, $p < .001$). Finally, difficulty making decisions tended to correlate with difficulty getting started once a decision has been made to do something ($r = .51$, $p < .001$).

The 25 items from the pilot version of the CDRS-SR that met the frequency and redundancy criteria and the two aforementioned additional items resulted in a 27-item final version of the CDRS-SR. The content validity of the CDRS-SR items is supported by their overlap with DSM-IV criteria for dysthymic disorder, the atypical features specifier, and the alternative research criterion B for dysthymic disorder.

The rank order of mean severity ratings of CDRS-SR items is depicted in Table 5.2, with 1 indicating minimal or absent symptoms and 4 being the rating associated with greatest severity. The six items that patients rated as most severe were depressed mood, worry, low energy, hopelessness, irritability, and poor self-esteem. The six items that patients rated as least severe included emotional responsivity, rejection sensitivity, ability to derive pleasure, difficulty getting started, adjusting to new circumstances, and suicidal ideation. The rank order of severity ratings of CDRS-SR items may yield important information about the patient's experience of dysthymia, as distinct from an interviewer's rating of symptom severity. Such rank ordering may also serve to objectify and prioritize areas to be addressed in psychotherapy or monitored for response to antidepressant medication.

## Summary

The CDRS is a 20-item clinician-rated scale that was developed to assess symptom severity and response to treatment in adult outpatients with dysthymic disorder by integrating *a priori* hypotheses regarding symptomatology and clinical course. Data were collected prior to treatment from participants in an ongoing drug treatment study of dysthymia. Frequency distributions and correlations were obtained for 43 clinician-rated items derived from the HRSD and the DSM-III criteria for dysthymic disorder. Infrequently endorsed and redundant items were eliminated. A 20-item CDRS with anchor points describing frequency and severity of symptoms was thereby generated.

**TABLE 5.2. Severity of Symptoms Endorsed on the CDRS-SR by Patients with Dysthymic Disorder**

| Rank order | Item number | Variable | Mean | Standard deviation | Minimum | Maximum |
|---|---|---|---|---|---|---|
| 1 | 1 | Mood | 3.36 | .80 | 1 | 4 |
| 2 | 15 | Worry | 3.07 | .91 | 1 | 4 |
| 3 | 3 | Low energy | 2.94 | .94 | 1 | 4 |
| 4 | 11 | Hopelessness | 2.93 | .97 | 1 | 4 |
| 6 | 9 | Irritability | 2.72 | .92 | 1 | 4 |
| 7 | 4 | Self-esteem | 2.67 | .98 | 1 | 4 |
| 8 | 19 | Assertiveness | 2.62 | .95 | 1 | 4 |
| 9 | 10 | Mood reactivity | 2.53 | 1.02 | 1 | 4 |
| 10 | 2 | Sleep | 2.52 | 1.13 | 1 | 4 |
| 11 | 14 | Self-pity | 2.47 | .94 | 1 | 4 |
| 12 | 6 | Concentration | 2.45 | .86 | 1 | 4 |
| 13 | 20 | Relationships | 2.44 | 1.05 | 1 | 4 |
| 14 | 12 | Tearfulness | 2.38 | 1.03 | 1 | 4 |
| 15 | 23 | Trust | 2.37 | .83 | 1 | 4 |
| 16 | 18 | Guilt | 2.27 | 1.05 | 1 | 4 |
| 17 | 5 | Productivity | 2.15 | .88 | 1 | 4 |
| 17 | 17 | Libido | 2.15 | 1.19 | 1 | 4 |
| 18 | 16 | Decisiveness | 1.93 | .90 | 1 | 4 |
| 20 | 7 | Sociability | 1.89 | .92 | 1 | 4 |
| 21 | 13 | Suicidality | 1.87 | .93 | 1 | 4 |
| 21 | 21 | Flexibility | 1.85 | .78 | 1 | 4 |
| 22 | 25 | Delayed response | 1.85 | .78 | 1 | 4 |
| 23 | 8 | Capacity for pleasure | 1.84 | .71 | 1 | 4 |
| 26 | 22 | Rejection sensitivity | 1.71 | .79 | 1 | 4 |
| 27 | 24 | Emotional responsivity | 1.66 | .76 | 1 | 4 |

*Note*. Higher scores indicate greater symptom severity. $n = 62$.

Comparison studies were conducted using CDRS and HRSD ratings from 108 participants in two drug treatment studies of dysthymia. The CDRS showed greater breadth in the range of individual item and sum scores than did the HRSD in a sample of dysthymics rated with both scales. This finding suggests that the CDRS may be more sensitive than the HRSD when measuring the milder symptoms of dysthymic disorder. Analyses conducted in patients rated before and after treatment showed that the CDRS performed well in measuring change during treatment. Correlations with response status indicated that the CDRS performed adequately as a change measure in this sample. ROC curves used to determine optimal cutoffs on the CDRS for response and nonresponse identified a CDRS score of 20 as having both high sensitivity and specificity to response status.

The CDRS-SR is a 27-item self-administered scale that was developed to assess symptom severity and response to treatment in adult outpatients with dysthymic disorder. Each item has four gradations of severity relevant to dysthymia. A grid format was chosen for the CDRS-SR to facilitate identification of omitted items or invalid response sets. Items contained in the CDRS-SR were empirically derived to reflect characteristic symptomatology endorsed by an outpatient sample meeting diagnostic criteria for dysthymic disorder. These 27 items represent all of the DSM-IV criteria for dysthymic disorder as well as the atypical features specifier and alternative research criterion B for dysthymic disorder presented in DSM-IV. Thus, the content validity of the empirically determined CDRS-SR items is supported by their overlap with DSM-IV criteria for dysthymic disorder.

## Acknowledgments

Preparation of this chapter was supported by U. S. Public Health Service Grant Nos. R01-37103 from the National Institute of Mental Health and M01-RR 00047 from the Division of Research Resources, National Institutes of Health. A portion of this chapter appeared in Mason, Kocsis, et al. (1993). 

## References

American Psychiatric Association. (1980). *Diagnostic and statistical manual of mental disorders* (3rd ed.). Washington, DC: Author.

American Psychiatric Association. (1994). *Diagnostic and statistical manual of mental disorders* (4th ed.). Washington, DC: Author.

Beck, A., Ward, C., Mendelson, M., Mock, J., & Erbaugh, J. (1961). An inventory for measuring depression. *Archives of General Psychiatry, 4*, 53–63.

Endicott, J., & Spitzer, R. L. (1979). Use of the Research Diagnostic Criteria and the Schedule for Affective Disorders and Schizophrenia to study affective disorders. *American Journal of Psychiatry, 136*, 52–56.

Endicott, J., Spitzer, R. L., Fleiss, J. L., & Cohen, J. (1976). The Global Assessment Scale: A procedure for measuring the overall severity of psychiatric disturbance. *Archives of General Psychiatry, 33*, 346–349.

Hamilton, M. (1960). A rating scale for depression. *Journal of Neurology, Neurosurgery, and Psychiatry, 25*, 56–62.

Hsiao, J. K., Bartko, J. J., & Potter, W. Z. (1989). Diagnosing diagnoses: Receiver operating characteristic methods and psychiatry. *Archives of General Psychiatry, 46*, 664–667.

Keller, M. B., Hirschfeld, R. M. A., Klein, D. N., Kocsis, J. H., McCullough, J. P., Miller, I., First, M., Holzer, C. P., Keitner, G. I., Marin, D. B., Shea, M. T. (in press). DSM-IV Mood Disorders Field Trial investigation results. *American Journal of Psychiatry.*

Kocsis, J. H., & Frances, A. J. (1987). A critical discussion of DSM-III Dysthymic Disorder. *American Journal of Psychiatry, 144*, 1534–1542.

Kocsis, J. H., Frances, A. J., Voss, C., Mann, J. J., Mason, B. J., & Sweeney, J. (1988). Imipramine treatment for chronic depression. *Archives of General Psychiatry, 45*, 253–257.

Mason, B. J., Kocsis, J. H., Leon, A. C., Thompson, S., Frances, A. J., Morgan, R. O., & Parides, M. K. (1993). Measurement of severity and treatment response in dysthymia. *Psychiatric Annals, 23*, 625–631.

Mason, B. J., Markowitz, J. C., & Klerman, G. L. (1993). IPT for dysthymic disorder. In G. L. Klerman & M. M. Weissman (Eds.), *New application of interpersonal psychotherapy* (pp. 225–264). Washington, DC: American Psychiatric Press.

Spitzer, R. L., Endicott, J., & Robins, E. (1978). *Research Diagnostic Criteria (RDC) for a selected group of functional disorders.* New York: New York State Psychiatric Institute.

Spitzer, R. L., & Williams, J. B. (1985). *Structured Clinical Interview for DSM-III.* New York: Biometrics Research Department, New York State Psychiatric Institute.

Zung, W. K. (1965). A self-rating depression scale. *Archives of General Psychiatry, 12*, 63–70.

CHAPTER SIX

# Social and Occupational Adjustment in Chronic Depression

RICHARD A. FRIEDMAN

In recent years clinicians and researchers have become increasingly aware that both acute and chronic depression are often associated with significant impairment in social and interpersonal functioning (Cassano, Perugi, Maremmani, & Akiskal, 1990; Weissman & Klerman, 1977; Weissman, Prusoff, Thompson, Harding, & Myers, 1978). In addition to the well-known affective, cognitive, and vegetative symptoms, depression is also characterized by significant disruption in the individual's capacity to work; to relate to spouse, family, and friends; and to enjoy leisure time. Social and occupational impairments vary widely, from the generally milder dysfunction in dysthymia to the often disabling functional impairments in acute major depression.

Recent estimates of the economic burden of depression on the national level underscore the extent of the social and occupational dysfunction of depression. For example, it is estimated that the cost of major depression in the U.S. work force is more than 172 million days yearly based on a 6-month prevalence rate of 5% for major depression (Dew, Bromet, Schulberg, Parkinson, & Curtis, 1991). In a recent study, Greenberg, Stiglin, Finkelstein, and Berndt (1993) estimated the annual cost of depression (major depression, bipolar disorder, and dysthymia) to be $43.7 billion. On the basis of an estimated rate of workplace impairment for depressed individuals of 20%, Greenberg et al. estimated the annual loss of productivity due to dysthymia alone to be approximately $9 billion.

This chapter addresses the specific social impairments in chronic depression and dysthymia, the effects of treatment on these impairments, and the clinical significance of social and occupational dysfunction in dysthymia. A better knowledge of the specific social areas that are impaired by depression will be helpful in guiding both treatment and rehabilitation of depressed patients.

## Assessment of Social Functioning in Depression

Assessment of a patient's social adjustment was formally incorporated into the multiaxial system of DSM-III (American Psychiatric Association, 1980). DSM-III included Axis V as a measure of adaptive functioning, with ratings on a 7-point scale ranging from "grossly impaired" to "superior." In DSM-III-R (American Psychiatric Association, 1987) and DSM-IV (American Psychiatric Association, 1994) Axis V was modified to the Global Assessment of Functioning Scale (GAFS), which assesses "psychological, social, and occupational functioning." The GAFS is a 90-point scale that combines assessments of social, occupational, and psychological functioning and represents a modification of the Global Assessment Scale (GAS) (Endicott, Spitzer, Fleiss, & Cohen, 1976). Since the GAFS includes symptom severity as well as indicators of social and occupational functioning, it is not an instrument that solely assesses social adjustment.

Recent interest in the social functioning aspect of affective illness has driven the development of specific instruments to assess social adjustment. A recent review lists at least 15 scales, which differ in terms of breadth of domains of functioning addressed, inclusion of symptoms, target population, and method of rating, that is, self- versus clinician-rated (Goldman, Skodol, & Lave, 1992). One of the most widely used scales is the Social Adjustment Scale–Self-Report (SAS-SR), which has demonstrated good reliability and validity (Weissman & Bothwell, 1976); its self-report ratings of adjustment correlate well with both clinician and spouse assessments.

Self-report scales are simple and inexpensive to administer. The SAS-SR covers five major areas of social functioning: work, as a worker, student, or housewife; social and leisure activities; relationships with extended family; parental role; and marital role. In each area, objective aspects of patient behavior and patient feelings are assessed during a 2-week period on a scale of 1 to 5, where higher scores reflect poorer functioning. The evaluations of the five areas are combined in a final overall adjustment score. The SAS-SR has been used to assess social adjustment in a community sample of normal controls, which serves as a useful comparison group to various patient samples (Weissman et al., 1978).

The use of a self-report instrument to assess social dysfunction in depressed patients may involve important limitations. The impact of depression on a patient's own assessment of his or her feelings and actual performance can be significant. For example, Morgado, Smith, Lecrubier, & Widlocher (1991) have shown that patients with major depression tend to report poor social adjustment, including both subjective distress and "objective performance," during the acute illness and more positively reevaluate it when in remission. Morgado et al. assessed social functioning with the clinician-rated Structured and Scaled Interview to Assess Maladjustment (SSIAM) (Gurland, Yorkston, Stone, Frank, & Fleiss, 1972). This study demonstrates that acutely depressed patients report poorer functioning than they do when in remission but does not clarify the question of whether the patients' reports of their functioning, in either the acute or remitted state, are objectively accurate inasmuch as the study did not use informants who could corroborate the patients' self-ratings. Weissman and Bothwell (1976) found excellent agreement between the patient's own social adjustment self-report rating (SAS-SR), a close informant's rating using the self-report form, and the clinician rating during interview. Finally, subjects who tend to falsify or who are delusional or semiliterate may give inaccurate self-ratings on an instrument such as the SAS-SR (Hogarty, 1973).

## Impact of Depression on Social Adjustment

The majority of studies of social and occupational impairment in depression have focused on patients with episodic major depression or on combined samples of acute and chronic depressives; there are few studies of patients with pure dysthymia or chronic depression.

Studies of social adjustment in depressed patients consistently show that they tend to be more socially impaired than psychiatrically healthy controls. Weissman compared the social adjustment of acutely depressed outpatients with community normal controls, alcoholics, and outpatient schizophrenics and found that depressives are more impaired than normals in all five of the following role areas: work, social leisure, extended family, marital, and parental. Depressives had the highest overall social impairment, followed next by the alcoholics and then by the outpatient schizophrenics (Weissman et al., 1978).

De Lisio reported in a study of 176 depressed outpatients (52% major depression, 10% bipolar, 38% dysthymic) that patients have broad social deficits that increase with severity of depression, that the areas of work and social leisure are the most disturbed, and that dysthymic patients, compared to unipolar depressives, have more overall social impairment because of greater disturbance in work and family domains. Furthermore, De Lisio noted that the observed social impairments are specific for primary depressive illness, since patients with panic disorder show relatively few social deficits compared to the depressed patients (De Lisio et al., 1986).

There are few significant correlations between sociodemographic characteristics and social impairment reported in the literature. In a study of dysthymic patients ($N$ = 110) Friedman, Parides, and Kocsis (1994) found no significant relationship between social functioning, as measured by the SAS-SR, and age, sex, race, educational or vocational level, or marital status. Weissman and Stewart both reported that younger depressed patients are more impaired. Weissman also noted that depressed females have significantly more impairment in the family unit role than depressed men (Stewart et al., 1988; Weissman et al., 1978).

## Depressive Severity, Chronicity, and Double Depression: Effects on Social Adjustment

There is good evidence that social impairment increases with increasing severity and chronicity of depression. Several studies report a strong correlation between depressive symptoms, as measured by the Hamilton Rating Scale for Depression (HRSD), and social impairment (De Lisio et al., 1986; Goldman et al., 1992;

Weissman et al., 1978). Friedman et al. (1994) found that overall social adjustment, as well as all individual domains of the SAS-SR, is significantly correlated with depressive severity, as measured by the HRSD, in a group of 110 dysthymic patients.

In a 6-month follow-up study, Klein (Klein, Taylor, Harding, & Dickstein, 1988) found that patients with double depression (major depression and dysthymia) have significantly greater overall social impairment compared to those with episodic major depression, although the study did not report on specific areas of social functioning. In that study, double depressives also reported poorer adolescent adjustment compared to episodic depressives, suggesting that chronic depression is associated with greater long-standing, as well as current, social impairment. Stewart (Stewart et al., 1988) reported that the more chronically depressed patients are more likely to rate themselves as functioning poorly than are those with less chronic illness.

Stewart et al. (1988) reported that patients with double depression have significantly worse overall social impairment than patients with dysthymia. Klein (1989) also noted an increase in social dysfunction associated with the occurrence of major depression in a sample of dysthymic patients. Neither study noted whether or not there are various types of social impairments that may be specific to major depression or dysthymia and that might distinguish one disorder from the other. Friedman et al. (1994) found that double depressives report significantly greater overall social dysfunction, as well as greater impairment in the leisure and financial domains, as measured by the SAS-SR, than do patients with pure dysthymia.

## Comorbidity and Social Adjustment

The effect of comorbid psychiatric disorders on social adjustment in chronic depression has received little attention. Bronisch and Hecht (1990) compared the social functioning of a group of patients with major depression ($n$ = 22) to that of patients with major depression and a comorbid anxiety disorder ($n$ = 20). They found no significant difference in social adjustment between the two groups, although the patients with major depression and anxiety disorder reported less close social support than those with pure major depression. Friedman et al. (1994) found that neither comorbid anxiety disorder nor personality disorder had a significant effect on social adjustment in a group of 110 patients with dysthymia.

## Treatment Effects on Social Impairment in Depression

Treatment has been shown to improve the social dysfunction of patients with acute forms of depression. Weissman et al. reported the differential effects of interpersonal psychotherapy (IPT) and amitriptyline (AMI) in two studies. The first study, which compared AMI versus IPT versus a combination of the two, found that patients in the psychotherapy groups show better social adjustment at the end of 8 but not 4 months of treatment (Weissman et al., 1974). The second study was a 1-year follow-up of acutely depressed patients who received 16 weeks of treatment with AMI, IPT, or a combination of both (Weissman, Klerman, Prusoff, Sholomskas, & Padian, 1981). It was found that patients who received psychotherapy alone or in combination with an antidepressant do significantly better on some measures of social functioning (i.e., work performance, communication, and interpersonal friction) than those who received pharmacotherapy alone. The authors concluded that psychotherapy is superior to medication in its effect on social impairment in the period following resolution of acute depression and that the differential treatment effect is evident only after a period of time.

In the National Institute of Mental Health Treatment of Depression Collaborative Research Program, the effectiveness of the following four treatments was compared in patients with major depression: IPT, cognitive-behavioral therapy (CBT), imipramine plus clinical management, and placebo plus clinical management. The authors used the GAS, which reflects both symptoms and functional impairment. The authors found significant improvement in GAS scores at the end of 16 weeks of treatment for all four treatment groups. When the sample was split into patients with more severe (GAS < 50) versus less severe (GAS > 50) functional impairment, there were significant differences between the treatments in their impact on functional impairment in the subgroup with severe impairment: Patients with severe functional impairment who were treated with imipramine had the greatest improvement in GAS scores; less improvement was associated with IPT and CBT, and least with placebo (Elkin et al., 1989).

Mintz, Mintz, Arruda, and Hwang (1992) reviewed 10 major studies of treatment of depression, involving mainly unipolar depressed patients, and found that work outcomes improved as the duration of treatment increased, with a maximum effect at 4 to 6 months. This lag in work recovery contrasted with the relatively quick response of depressive symptoms to treatment regardless of whether the study involved short-term drug treatment (4 to 6 weeks), brief psychotherapy (10 to 16 weeks), or maintenance therapy over a 6 to 9 month period. These results are consistent with the 8-month maintenance study that reported that improvement in social functioning took 6 to 8 months to occur (Weissman et al., 1974).

The impact of treatment on social impairment in patients with dysthymia and chronic depression contrasts with that in patients with episodic major depression. Kocsis concluded in a double-blind study comparing imipramine to placebo (Kocsis, Frances, & Voss, 1988; Kocsis, Frances, Voss, et al., 1988) that responders to treatment at 6 weeks show significant improvement in overall social functioning compared to nonresponders, although few patients achieved a level of social adjustment comparable to Weissman's (1978) community normal controls. The imipramine-treated group showed improvement in most areas of social functioning, including work, family, and marital domains.

Stewart et al. (1988) also reported that patients who responded to treatment in a 6-week double-blind trial of phenelzine, imipramine, or placebo reported significantly improved social functioning compared to nonresponders. Stewart also noted that while responders clearly were functioning better than nonresponders, after 6 weeks of treatment only 28% of responders rated themselves as well as or better than the mean of social functioning for Weissman's (1978) community controls.

Agosti, Stewart, and Quitkin (1991) reported similar findings in a 6-week placebo-controlled double-blind study of phenelzine, imipramine, and L-deprenyl in a sample of 61 depressed outpatients (25% with major depression, 31% dysthymia, 44% double depression): 60% of responders who started with "poor" functioning improved to "good" functioning. The fact that many of the patients who responded to pharmacotherapy in the aforementioned studies still reported significant social impairment may reflect the relatively short (6 weeks) duration of treatment; 6 weeks of antidepressant treatment may not be long enough to see the maximal effect of treatment on social adjustment.

Several authors have noted that certain domains of social and occupational functioning may recover or change differentially with treatment. For example, De Lisio et al. (1986) and Cassano et al. (1990) reported that enjoyment of leisure time remains markedly impaired even after significant improvement in depressive symptoms and other areas of social functioning such as work, relationships with family and spouse, and sexual adjustment. In contrast, Friedman et al. (1994) found a significant improvement in leisure activities in dysthymic patients whose depression responded to 10 weeks of open desipramine treatment compared to nonresponders. These divergent findings may reflect, in part, the fact that both the De Lisio and Cassano studies used mixed samples of patients, the majority of whom had acute depression.

Thus, in some chronically depressed patients, antidepressants are effective in treating social dysfunction as well as symptoms of depression. From a theoretical standpoint, such results may help to elucidate the nature of the disorder. If the social impairments in chronic depression were the signs of a personality disorder, one would not predict that social functioning would improve as depression lifted. The observed improvement in the patients in the studies cited earlier suggests that for some dysthymic and chronically depressed patients social impairment is a symptom of a mood disorder rather than a result of underlying character pathology. Furthermore, the rapid improvement in social adjustment seen in some dysthymics with acute treatment (6 weeks) suggests that social dysfunction may be a state-related abnormality of chronic depression.

## Long-Term Treatment Effects on Social Dysfunction in Chronic Depression

Effects of longer-term treatment on social adjustment in chronic depression and dysthymia remain unclear. In a 3-month follow-up study, Perugi, Maremmani, McNair, Cassano, and Akiskal (1988) studied the social dysfunction of 99 depressed outpatients (79% were unipolar, 8% bipolar, and 13% dysthymic) and found that work and leisure areas were the most affected. They reported that work impairment was related to severity of symptoms but that impairment in leisure activities persisted despite improvement in depressive symptoms. The authors proposed that the deficit in leisure function may represent a trait marker of depression. Given the short follow-up period, it was not possible to determine whether impairment in leisure activities represented a trait marker of depression or simply a residual symptom of partially treated depression. Furthermore, Perugi et al. studied a group of patients most of whom had acute depression. Their findings were consistent with those from studies of acute depressives (Mintz et al., 1992), namely, that there is a significant delay between the early improvement of depressive symptoms and the subsequent improvement in social functioning.

Bauwens, Tracy, Pardoen, vander Elst, and Mendewicz (1991) addressed this question in a study of social adjustment in bipolar and unipolar depressed patients who were in remission for at least 6 months. They found that both patient groups had mild social maladjustment relative to normal controls, particularly in the area of social and leisure activities. Bauwen's data were consistent with other studies that reported varying degrees of social dysfunction in remitted patients with episodic major depression (Bothwell & Weissman, 1977; Weissman et al., 1981).

It should be noted that since the studies of Perugi and Bauwnes involved mainly patients with acute unipolar or bipolar depression, the results may not generalize to patients with chronic forms of depression.

In the longest follow-up of chronically depressed patients to date, Kocsis, Sutton, and Frances (1991) assessed 25 dysthymic patients an average of 3.5 years after participation in 6-week imipramine trial. They found that 89% of imipramine responders met criteria for recovery at follow-up compared with 31% in the comparison groups of nonresponders or noncompleters. Responders, two-thirds of whom were still on medication at follow-up, also showed superior social adjustment compared to the other groups, with a level of function close to Wiessman's (1978) community controls. While the sample is small, these data suggest that longer-term treatment with antidepressant medication can lead both to sustained recovery from depressive symptoms and reversal of social dysfunction in patients with chronic depression.

## Conclusion

Chronic depression and dysthymia produce considerable social and occupational impairment, reducing the quality of life experienced by sufferers. Affected individuals may have varying degrees of impairment in major social roles involved in work, family life, intimate relationships, and social and leisure time. Aside from individual morbidity, chronic depression and dysthymia exact significant costs from society: The annual cost attributed to decreased productive potential at the workplace from dysthymia alone has been estimated at $9 billion.

Social dysfunction tends to increase with greater chronicity and severity of depression. There is strong evidence that short-term tricyclic and monoamine oxidase inhibitor (MAOI) antidepressant treatment can significantly improve social dysfunction as well as alleviate depressive symptoms in patients who respond to pharmacotherapy. This suggests that for some patients social dysfunction is a treatable symptom of a mood disorder rather than a result of character pathology.

Whether longer-term treatment of patients with chronic depression will result in recovery of normal social functioning, in contrast to more moderate improvement in functioning, is unclear at present. Limited but encouraging evidence suggests that adequate pharmacotherapy can both produce sustained recovery from depressive symptoms and lead to reversal of social impairment in patients with chronic depression (Kocsis et al., 1991), but this finding needs verification.

Several other issues related to social adjustment in dysthymia deserve mention. Most studies of social adjustment in depression to date have involved heterogeneous diagnostic samples. Larger studies of patients with pure dysthymia and double depression are needed to more clearly determine the exact types of social impairments in dysthymia and to contrast them to those in other forms of depression. There is conflicting preliminary evidence from studies of depressed patients as to whether or not some areas of social functioning show a differential response pattern to treatment (e.g., whether enjoyment of leisure time remains impaired when other social areas show improvement), a matter that requires further study. The relationship between social dysfunction and the course of depression needs to be better understood; for example, we need to know if mild social impairments during remission increase the risk of recurrent depression. The relationship between premorbid social adjustment and subsequent functioning during depression needs clarification.

The potential efficacy of the newer serotonin-selective reuptake inhibitors such as fluoxetine and sertraline in treating social dysfunction in chronically depressed patients remains to be studied. The role of various psychotherapies in treating social dysfunction in dysthymia and chronic depression has received little attention. Given the effectiveness of IPT in treating the social dysfunction in patients with acute depression (Weissman et al., 1974), there is a rationale for controlled trials of IPT and other psychotherapies in chronically depressed patients.

Clinicians need to be aware that social and occupational dysfunction, like the well-known affective and vegetative symptomatology, is both common and often treatable in patients with chronic depression and dysthymia. Given the profound impact of depression on the individual quality of life, as well as the national economic burden of depression, the various social impairments must remain an important focus of the clinician as newer treatments for chronic depression and dysthymia emerge.

## Acknowledgment

This chapter is adapted from Friedman (1993). Copyright 1993 by Slack, Inc. Adapted by permission.

## References

Agosti, V., Stewart, J. W., & Quitkin, F. M. (1991). Life satisfaction and psychosocial functioning in chronic depression: Effect of acute treatment with antidepressants. *Journal of Affective Disorders, 23*, 35–41.

American Psychiatric Association. (1980). *Diagnostic and statistical manual of mental disorders* (3rd ed.). Washington, DC: Author.

American Psychiatric Association. (1987). *Diagnostic and statistical manual of mental disorders* (3rd ed., rev.). Washington, DC: Author.

American Psychiatric Association. (1994). *Diagnostic and statistical manual of mental disorders* (4th ed.). Washington, DC: Author.

Bauwens, F., Tracy, A., Pardoen, D., vander Elst, M., & and Mendewicz, J. (1991). Social adjustment of remitted bipolar and unipolar out-patients: A comparison with age- and sex-matched controls. *British Journal of Psychiatry, 159*, 239–244.

Bothwell, S., & Weissman, M. M. (1977). Social impairments four years after an acute depressive episode. *American Journal of Orthopsychiatry, 47*, 231–237.

Bronisch, T., & Hecht, H. (1990). Major depression with and without a coexisting anxiety disorder: Social dysfunction, social integration, and personality features. *Journal of Affective Disorders, 20*, 151–157.

Cassano, G. B., Perugi, G., Maremmani, I., & Akiskal, H. S. (1990). Social adjustment in dysthymia. In S. W. Burton & H. S. Akiskal (Eds.), *Dysthymic disorder* (pp. 78–85). Washington, DC: American Psychiatric Press.

De Lisio, G., Maremmani, I., Perugi, G., Cassano, G. B., Deltito, J., & Akiskal, H. S. (1986). Impairment of work and leisure in depressed outpatients. Journal of Affective Disorders, *10*, 79–84.

Dew, M. A., Bromet, E. J., Schulberg, H. C., Parkinson, D. K., & Curtis, E. C. (1991). Factors affecting service utilization for depression in a white-collar population. *Social Psychiatry and Psychiatric Epidemiology, 26*, 230–237.

Elkin, I., Shea, T., Watkins, J. T., Imber, S. D., Sotsky, S. M., Collins, J. F., Glass, D. R., Pilkonis, P. A., Leber, W. R., Docherty, J. P., Fiester, S. J., & Parloff, M. B. (1989). National Institute of Mental Health Treatment of Depression Collaborative Research Program. *Archives of General Psychiatry, 46*, 971–982.

Endicott, J., Spitzer, R. L., Fleiss, J. L., & Cohen, J. (1976). The Global Assessment Scale: A procedure for measuring overall severity of psychiatric disturbance. *Archives of General Psychiatry, 33*, 766–771.

Friedman, R. A. (1993). Social impairment in dysthymnia. *Psychiatric Annals, 23*, 632–637.

Friedman, R. A., Parides, M., Kocsis, J. H. (1994). *The clinical significance of social dysfunction in chronic depression*. Unpublished manuscript, Department of Psychiatry, Cornell University Medical College.

Goldman, H. H., Skodol, A. E., & Lave, T. R. (1992). Revising Axis V for DSM-IV: A review of measures of social functioning. *American Journal of Psychiatry, 149*, 1148–1156.

Greenberg, P. E., Stiglin, L. E., Finkelstein, S. N., & Berndt, E. R. (1993).

The economic burden of depression in 1990. *Journal of Clinical Psychiatry, 54*, 405–418.

Gurland, B. J., Yorkston, N. J., Stone, A. R., Frank, J. D., & Fleiss, J. L. (1972). The Structured and Scaled Interview to Assess Maladjustment (SSIAM): I. Description, rationale, and development. *Archives of General Psychiatry, 27*, 264–267.

Hogarty, J. (1973). Informant rating of community adjustment. In I. E. Waskow & M. B. Parloff (Eds.), *Psychotherapy change measures: Report of Clinical Research Branch, National Institute of Mental Health, Outcome Measures Project* (Publication No. 8DM74-120). Washington, DC: U.S. Government Printing Office.

Klein, D. N. (1989). Social adjustment in affective disorders [letter]. *American Journal of Psychiatry, 146*, 1086–1087.

Klein, D. N., Taylor, E. B., Harding, K., & Dickstein, S. (1988). Double depression and episodic major depression: Demographic, clinical, familial, personality, and socioenvironmental characteristics and short-term outcome. *American Journal of Psychiatry, 145*, 1226–1231.

Kocsis, J. H., Frances, A. J., & Voss, C. (1988). Imipramine for treatment of chronic depression. *Archives of General Psychiatry, 45*, 253–257.

Kocsis, J. H., Frances, A. J., Voss, C., Mason, B. J., Mann, J. J., & Sweeney, J. (1988). Imipramine and sociovocational adjustment in chronic depression. *American Journal of Psychiatry, 145*, 997–999.

Kocsis, J. H., Sutton, B. M., & Frances, A. J. (1991). Long-term follow-up of chronic depression treated with imipramine. *Journal of Clinical Psychiatry, 52*, 56–59.

Mintz, J., Mintz, L. I., Arruda, M. J., & Hwang, S. S. (1992). Treatments of depression and the functional capacity to work. *Archives of General Psychiatry, 49*, 761–768.

Morgado, A., Smith, M., Lecrubier, Y., & Widlocher, D. (1991). Depressed subjects unwittingly overreport poor social adjustment which they reappraise when recovered. *Journal of Nervous and Mental Disease, 179*, 614–619.

Perugi, G., Maremmani, I., McNair, D. M., Cassano, G. B., & Akiskal, H. S. (1988). Differential changes in areas of social adjustment from depressive episodes through recovery. *Journal of Affective Disorders, 15*, 39–43.

Stewart, J. W., Quitkin, F. M., McGrath, P. J., Rabkin, J. G., Markowitz, J. C., Tricamo, E., & Klein, D. F. (1988). Social functioning in chronic depression: Effect of 6 weeks of antidepressant treatment. *Psychiatry Research, 25*, 213–222.

Weissman, M. M., & Bothwell, S. (1976). Assessment of social adjustment by patient self-report. *Archives of General Psychiatry, 33*, 1111–1115.

Weissman, M. M., & Klerman, G. L. (1977). The chronic depressive in the community: Unrecognized and poorly treated. *Comprehensive Psychiatry, 18*, 523–532.

Weissman, M. M., Klerman, G. L., Paykel, E. S., et al. (1974). Treatment effects on the social adjustment of depressed patients. *Archives of General Psychiatry, 30*, 771–778.

Weissman, M. M., Klerman, G. L., Prusoff, B. A., Sholomskas, D., & Padian, N. (1981). Depressed outpatients: Results one year after treatment with drugs and/or interpersonal therapy. *Archives of General Psychiatry, 38*, 51–55.

Weissman, M. M., Prusoff, B. A., Thompson, W. D., Harding, P. S., & Myers, J. K. (1978). Social adjustment by self-report in a community sample and in psychiatric outpatients. *Journal of Nervous and Mental Disease, 166*, 317–326.

CHAPTER SEVEN

# Family and Genetic Epidemiologic Studies

DANIEL W. GOODMAN
JOHN BARNHILL

The inclusion of dysthymic disorder as an Axis I mood disorder was one of the more controversial shifts in psychiatric nosology represented by DSM-III (American Psychiatric Association, 1980; Kocsis & Frances, 1987). While DSM-III, DSM-III-R (American Psychiatric Association, 1987), and DSM-IV (American Psychiatric Association, 1994) have highlighted the relationship between dysthymia and the major affective disorders, some prominent theoreticians have argued that at least some chronic depressions should be viewed as related more to the personality disorders (Frances, 1980; Frances & Cooper, 1981). On the basis of clinical features, other investigators have questioned the validity of dysthymia as a distinct diagnostic entity (Angst & Wicki, 1991). Dysthymics have high lifetime rates of comorbidity with major depression, and dysthymia without any comorbid diagnoses is rare in most studies (Markowitz, Moran, Kocsis, & Frances, 1992; Weissman, Leaf, Bruce, & Florio, 1988).

## Family Studies

Family data provide a means of addressing the aforementioned issues. A relationship between dysthymia and the mood disorders could be confirmed if probands with dysthymia are found to have elevated family rates of mood disorders or, alternatively, if probands with other mood disorders are found to have elevated family rates of dysthymia. Strongest evidence for this hypothesis would come from comparing relatives of probands with pure dysthymia without comorbid mood disorders (or, ideally, with no comorbid diagnoses of any sort) to relatives of probands with no psychiatric illness, since coexisting illnesses in the probands could influence the diagnoses in relatives. A similar approach using family data could help clarify the nature of the relationship between dysthymia and personality disorders. Furthermore, family data can also shed light on the validity of dysthymia as a distinct diagnostic entity independent of other mood or personality disorders. One approach to establishing the validity of a diagnostic category is to examine whether or not it is specifically transmitted within families (Robins & Guze, 1970). If dysthymia is found to "breed true"—that is, if relatives of dysthymic probands are more likely to have dysthymia independent of comorbid diagnoses—this specificity of transmission would provide support for the validity of dysthymia as a diagnostic category.

In addition to clarifying questions about the nosology of dysthymia, data from properly designed studies of families can help clarify the role of specific etiologic factors in dysthymia. Demonstration of familial aggregation of a disorder or disorders does not by itself identify whether genetic factors, environmental factors, or both are responsible for the aggregation (Weissman et al., 1986). Nonadoptive relatives share genes, but the family also provides the environment in which many influential nongenetic variables—both biological (diet, toxins, infections, etc.) and psychosocial—act. Major depression and dysthymia are both associated with significant social impairment that can impact directly on the family environment and may be a risk factor for psychiatric illness (Friedman, 1993). Specialized designs such as adoption or twin studies could explore the specific role of genetic factors in the etiology of dysthymia, and assessment of environmental variables could shed light on the role of the environment in the etiology of dysthymia. Studies applying these methods to dysthymia are, however, extremely limited. This review therefore focuses on extant family studies of chronic depression but also summarizes the results of studies that attempt to address the roles of genetic and environmental variables in the etiology of chronic depression.

## Early Efforts: Akiskal and Colleagues

In a seminal early effort to conceptualize chronic depression and to address questions regarding heterogeneity within the category of chronic depression, Akiskal, King, Rosenthal, Robinson, and Scott-Strauss (1981) reported on 137 consecutively evaluated chronic depressives who were referred to a mood clinic. In the course of assessing and treating these patients, they developed a classification of chronic depression based on clinical features and response to medication as follows: "subaffective dysthymics" (early onset, antidepressant responsive), "character-spectrum disorder" (early onset, antidepressant nonresponsive), "chronic primary unipolar depressives" (later onset, i.e., after age 25), and "chronic secondary depressives" (with a primary medical or nonaffective psychiatric disorder). Family history data were obtained for all first-degree relatives using the Family History–Research Diagnostic Criteria (FH-RDC). A sample of episodic unipolar depressives was included as a control group.

The character-spectrum group differed significantly from the other groups in that only 3% of the 30 patients reported a family history of depression. Subaffective dysthymics resembled chronic primary, chronic secondary, and episodic unipolar depressives in reports of family histories of depression (30%, 42%, 16%, and 20%, respectively). The subaffective dysthymics, however, stood out in that 35% of the 20 patients reported a family history of bipolar disorder compared to 5% or less for the other groups. Overall, the subaffective dysthymics and chronic unipolars most often reported a family history of any affective disorder (65% and 47% of 38 patients, respectively), with the character-spectrum subjects reporting this least often (6%) and the chronic secondary and episodic unipolars being intermediate (at 18% and 23%). The character-spectrum subjects also differed significantly from the other groups in more often reporting a family history of alcoholism (53% versus 10% to 29%), developmental object loss (60% versus 21% to 35%), and parental assortative mating for psychiatric illness (47% versus 10% to 31%). Rates for comorbid substance abuse were highest in this group as well (60%).

Akiskal's study thus emphasized several findings, most prominently the heterogeneous nature of chronic depressions. The high rate of family history of affective disorders in the subaffective dysthymics, higher than for any other group, is striking and suggests a strong connection with the affective disorders. The high rate of bipolar disorder in families of this group is a surprising finding. Equally noteworthy, however, are the remarkably low reports of affective disorders in the relatives of the character-spectrum patients. Akiskal concluded that the early-onset chronic depressions comprise two groups with presumed different etiologies, one related more to the personality disorders and the other to the affective disorders.

While Akiskal's study was an important pioneering effort to conceptualize the relationship between chronic depressions and the mood and personality disorders, the study lacked methodologic features that have more recently become standards for the conduct of family studies. Proband diagnoses were made clinically without the use of structured diagnostic assessments. Family history was obtained by raters who were not blind to proband diagnosis, and family data was obtained primarily from probands without direct assessments of relatives. Familial diagnoses were only reported by presence or absence of family history of a particular illness–using the family as a unit of analysis–without using statistical methodologies to analyze rates of illness within families as well. Given the high rates of comorbid substance abuse in the character-spectrum group and the elevated rates of depression that many studies have documented in families of substance abusers, the remarkably low rates of depressive disorders in the families of this group raise questions as to the reliability of these data. Cloninger, Reich, and Wetzel (1979) reported that 15% of adult first-degree relatives of probands with primary alcoholism have a history of depression. Using the family (as Akiskal did) rather than the individual relative (as did Cloninger) as the unit of analysis should result in higher rates. For example, Hesselbrock, Tennen, Stabinau, and Hesselbrock (1983) reported that 25% of nondepressed alcoholics have a family history of depression, with higher rates in families of depressed alcoholics.

## More Recent Studies: Klein and Colleagues

In more recent studies, Klein et al. have sought to explore the relationship of dysthymia to affective and personality disorders by using family history methodologies (Klein, Clark, Dansky, & Margolis, 1988; Klein, Riso, & Anderson, 1993; Klein, Taylor, Dickstein, & Harding, 1988). These studies benefited both from the formulation of dysthymic disorder in DSM-III and dysthymia in DSM-III-R and from advances in the design of family studies.

In one study, 32 primary early-onset dythymics and 35 primary nonbipolar nonchronic major depressives were compared on a number of characteristics including family history (Klein, Taylor, Dickstein, & Harding, 1988). As with Akiskal's study, family history data were obtained only from probands using FH-RDCs and by raters who were not blind to proband diagnoses. Of the primary early-onset dysthymics, 59% were in a major depressive episode at the time of the study. All but one of the dysthymics had a lifetime history of major depression.

Compared to nonchronic depressives, dysthymics reported significantly higher rates of family histories of nonbipolar depressive disorders (78% versus 54%), bipolar II disorder (19% versus 3%) but not bipolar I disorder, and antisocial personality disorder (22% versus 6%). Similarly, using the individual relative rather than the family as the unit of analysis, Klein et al. found that lifetime rates for a major affective disorder were significantly higher in the relatives of the dysthymic group (49% versus 29%).

Noting the high rates of affective disorders in relatives of dysthymics (the use of only family history and not direct interview data probably even resulted in an underestimate of these rates), Klein et al. suggested that early-onset dysthymia may not only be closely related to major affective illness but may be a more severe form than episodic major depression. At the same time, however, noting the higher comorbidity with borderline and/or schizotypal personality disorder in the dysthymic group (47% versus 14%) and the higher family histories of antisocial personality disorder, they also stated that the data were consistent with the view that early-onset dysthymia is related to the severe personality disorders. They concluded that it is unlikely that most forms of dysthymia are simply a consequence of primary personality disorders. However, this study did not fully resolve questions as to whether or not early-onset dysthymia (1) is a heterogeneous category with distinct, nonoverlapping characterologic and affective subgroups, as suggested by Akiskal; (2) is often associated with personality disorder features as a consequence of the deleterious impact of chronic depression on personality development; (3) is often associated with characterologic features owing to shared etiologic processes in the personality and affective disorders; or (4) appears to be associated with characterologic features that are in fact independent of the chronic depression but nonetheless frequently observed owing to factors such as referral bias (e.g., personality characteristics could contribute to the likelihood that a chronic depressive would be referred).

This study is consistent with Akiskal's in finding markedly high rates of affective disorders in relatives of early-onset dysthymics. Like Akiskal's, it suggests a familial relationship between dysthymia and bipolar disorder. However, as in Akiskal's study, the data on familial rates were limited by the use of only family history data obtained by raters who were not blind to proband diagnosis. Neither of these studies addressed questions about the course of illness in relatives, such as whether relatives of dysthymics were more likely to have episodic or chronic depressive disorders. Determining whether relatives of probands with dysthymia are more likely to have dysthymia, that is, evaluating the specificity of transmission of dysthymia, is important for establishing the nosologic status and validity of this diagnosis.

Finally, Klein's study is notable in that all but one of the 32 early-onset dysthymics had a lifetime history of major depressive disorder (MDD). The dysthymic group had an early average age (17.8 years) of onset of MDD. Early-onset major depressives have high familial rates of MDD (Weissman et al., 1984). Controlling for age of onset of MDD in the dysthymic and episodic depressive groups did not explain the higher family rates of MDD of the dysthymics, but this study could not clarify the degree to which dysthymia as a diagnosis independent of early-onset MDD was responsible for the high family rates of MDD. A pure dysthymia group, uncomplicated by MDD, would be needed to assess the contribution of dysthymia to familial risk for MDD. In addition, inclusion of a pure dysthymia group would be important in order to explore hypotheses about the heterogeneity of early-onset chronic depressions. For example, if pure dysthymia and dysthymia comorbid with MDD have distinct clinical features and familial rates of illnesses unexplained by the absence or presence of MDD, then dysthymia with and without MDD might represent distinct disorders and the concept of heterogeneity of chronic depressions would be supported.

A second study by Klein et al. further explored the question of familial links between dysthymia and unipolar MDD using direct interviews of relatives rather than family history data (Klein, Clark, Dansky, & Margolis, 1988; Klein et al., 1993). All adolescent and adult offspring (ages 14 to 22) of 24 unipolar depressive probands and of two control groups—one with medical conditions and one a screened normal community sample—were directly assessed for the presence of psychiatric illness by interviewers blind to parental diagnoses. Compared to offspring of the medical and normal controls, a significantly greater proportion of the offspring of unipolar probands met criteria for DSM-III dysthymic disorder and for DSM-III-R primary early-onset dysthymia. Klein et al. concluded that these findings supported the thesis that dysthymia is familially related to the major affective disorders. However, 33% (8 of 24) of the unipolar probands had an underlying chronic minor depression (an RDC diagnosis that closely resembles the DSM-III and DSM-III-R constructs of dysthymic disorder and dysthymia), while 8 of the 9 dysthymic offspring came from this subgroup of chronically depressed unipolar probands. These data are therefore also consistent with the hypothesis that parental dysthymia and not unipolar depression per se is responsible for dysthymia in the offspring. While failing therefore to establish clearly a familial link between unipolar MDD and dysthymia, this study provides some evidence that chronicity of depression may breed true, that is, transmit specifically within families.

## The Cornell Dysthymia Study

In the course of evaluating patients with chronic depressive disorders, Kocsis and colleagues in the Cornell Dysthymia Study obtained family history data using a modification of the FH-RDC. Unlike earlier studies, the sample included a significant number of pure dysthymics in addition to dysthymics with superimposed major depression (proband diagnoses were obtained with the Structured Clinical Interview for DSM-III-R [SCID]). Probands were queried about the presence of chronic and episodic depressive disorders and alcohol abuse in all adult first-degree relatives. Owing to the difficulty of using family history alone to accurately measure the severity and number of depressive symptoms, distinctions were not made between dysthymia, double depression, and chronic major depression, all of which were characterized as chronic depression. In contrast, relatives with either single or recurrent major depressions with subsequent remission and without a history of chronic depression were characterized as episodic depressives. Relatives could not receive lifetime diagnoses of both episodic and chronic depression. Family history data were not obtained blindly.

Data were collected on 360 adult first-degree relatives of 87 dysthymic patients. Of the dysthymic probands, 38% had no lifetime history of major depression (pure dysthymia) although other comorbid diagnoses could be present, and 62% were double depressives. The mean age of probands was 36.9 (*SD* = 9.6); 58% were female. There was a mean of 4.1 (*SD* = 1.9) relatives per proband, 62% were over age 40, and 51% were female. Pure dysthymics and double depressives did not differ in age, sex, or number of relatives per proband, and the relatives of these two proband groups were also identical with respect to sex and age distribution.

Pure dysthymics and double depressives both reported high rates of depressive disorders in relatives. Of the relatives of pure dysthymics, 27% had a history of a depressive disorder—11% were chronic depressives and 15% acute depressives. For the relatives of probands with double depression, 32% had a depressive diagnosis; of these, 20% were chronic depressives and 12% acute depressives. A history of alcohol abuse was reported for 18% of the relatives of pure dysthymics and 19% of the relatives of double depressives. Using the family unit rather than individual relatives as the basis of analysis, pure dysthymics and double depressives, respectively, reported high family histories of chronic depression (34% and 61%), acute depression (46% and 39%), and any depression (64% and 76%). Some probands had relatives with acute depression as well as relatives with chronic depression. A family history of alcohol abuse was reported for 46% of pure dysthymics and 54% of double depressives. Double depressives differed from pure dysthymics in having significantly higher rates of chronic depression in their relatives individually and in their families as a whole. In other respects, the two groups were similar.

Like Klein's study, the Cornell study shows high rates of depressive disorders in relatives of probands with double depression. Additionally, this sample provides evidence that pure dysthymia without comorbid major depression is also associated with high rates of affective disorders in relatives. However, an appropriate normal control group would be needed to be able to state most strongly that these data confirm a familial relationship between dysthymia and major depression. The Cornell probands had high rates of chronic (as well as acute) depression in their relatives, consistent with Klein's study of offspring of unipolar probands, but a control group of episodic depressives would be needed to establish whether or not chronic depression is specifically transmitted in families.

## Unresolved Issues

Taken together, these studies provide strong initial evidence of a relationship between dysthymia and major depression and for the placement of dysthymia within the Axis I mood disorders sections of DSM-III, DSM-III-R, and DSM-IV. A familial relationship between dysthymia and major depression is the most consistent finding. The relationship between dysthymia and the personality disorders remains unclear. Akiskal and Klein both found evidence for an association with personality disorders in a subset of their chronic depressives. However, comprehensive data on personality disorders in relatives of chronic depressives have been lacking. There are suggestions as well in these studies that dysthymia may aggregate specifically in families. However, family study data obtained by *direct* interview of relatives will be needed to confirm these findings and to assess more fully the relationship between major mood disorders, personality disorders, and dysthymia. Evaluating the validity of potential subcategories of chronic depressives will simultaneously require not only more comprehensive assessments of relatives but well-characterized distinct subgroups of probands who fit the proposed subcategories. Two family studies have begun to clarify some of these outstanding issues.

## Contemporary Studies: Goodman and Colleagues

In a recent study Goodman et al. (in press) examined DSM-III-R diagnoses of 435 directly interviewed adult first-degree relatives of

148 psychiatrically ill and 45 screened normal control probands. The data came from a family study of probands with (1) panic disorder without comorbid major depression; (2) panic disorder with comorbid major depression; and (3) early onset major depression without panic disorder (Weissman et al., 1993). Thirty-three of the psychiatrically ill probands also had comorbid dysthymia. The study methodology included all of the advances that have become standard in family studies, including blind assessments of relatives and "best estimate" diagnoses of subjects via clinical review of all available data, including direct interviews, family history data, and review of medical and psychiatric records.

Goodman et al. mainly addressed two questions. They examined the relationship between the primary proband diagnoses (panic disorder and/or major depression) and dysthymia in relatives to determine which other diagnoses may be related to dysthymia. Probands with comorbid dysthymia were excluded from these analyses in order to ensure that dysthymia in relatives could not be attributed to dysthymia in the probands. Early-onset major depression was associated with an approximately 4.5-fold increase in rates of dysthymia in relatives of probands compared to relatives of screened normal controls. Only nonsignificant increases in rates of dysthymia were noted in relatives of the other two proband groups (panic disorder with or without comorbid major depression).

Specificity of familial transmission of dysthymia ("breeding true") was tested by comparing rates of dysthymia in relatives of probands with and without dysthymia in each of the three psychiatrically ill proband groups. Increased rates of dysthymia were observed in relatives of dysthymic probands in all three of the ill proband groups, with no evidence for differences among the three proband groups in the strength of the association between dysthymia in probands and in relatives. Overall, dysthymia in probands was estimated to confer a 2.9-fold increased risk of dysthymia in relatives irrespective of the primary proband diagnosis.

Goodman's analysis thus provides strong evidence for a relationship between early onset major depression, a highly familial form of major depression, and dysthymia. In addition, the demonstration of specific familial aggregation of dysthymia provides further support for the concept of dysthymia as a valid diagnostic category that is distinct from but related to major depression.

However, because these data came from a family study that was primarily designed to explore the relationship between panic disorder and major depression, Goodman et al. were unable to explore the possibility that the concept of dysthymia subsumes a heterogeneous group of patients with differing characteristics. Although they did not find any significant differences in specificity of aggregation of dysthymia among proband groups, and thus no evidence that dysthymia with comorbid panic disorder differs from dysthymia with comorbid major depression, there was minimal power to test hypotheses regarding the heterogeneity of dysthymia inasmuch as there were only 33 dysthymic probands. The study thus left unaddressed, for example, questions as to whether early and late onset dysthymia, or dysthymia with comorbid major depression (double depression) and dysthymia alone (pure dysthymia), have different characteristics.

## Contemporary Studies: Klein and Colleagues

In the most comprehensive study to date, Klein et al. (1995) conducted a family study of 97 outpatients with early-onset dysthymia, 45 outpatients with episodic major depression, and 45 normal controls and their 882 first-degree relatives, approximately 40% of whom were directly interviewed. This study, which was specifically designed to study the relationship between early-onset dysthymia, major mood disorders, and personality disorders, was notable for its use of state-of-the-art assessments of both personality disorders and the more commonly measured Axis I disorders in probands and relatives. As with Goodman's study, the data were obtained using blind diagnostic assessments and "best estimate" diagnoses for both Axis I and Axis II disorders. Finally, the large sample of dysthymics provided some power to begin to explore the notion that early-onset dysthymia represents a heterogeneous disorder, as Akiskal first proposed.

Consistent with the results of other studies reported here, Klein et al. observed a familial association between dysthymia and major depression, with elevated rates of major depression in relatives of dysthymics compared to relatives of normal controls. The association appeared unidirectional in that relatives of episodic major depressives did not have increased rates of dysthymia compared to normals, although they did have increased rates of chronic major depression. This finding contrasts with the observation by Goodman et al. of increased rates of dysthymia in relatives of early onset major depressive probands who did not have comorbid dysthymia. However, Goodman's study did not distinguish carefully between dysthymia and chronic major depression in relatives. Combining these studies' patterns of familial aggregation is difficult owing to the lopsided associations between dysthymia and major depression, but, at a minimum, the data convincingly support the hypothesis of a familial relationship between dysthymia and major depression.

Klein et al. observed that relatives of dysthymics also had elevated rates of chronic depression (including both dysthymia and chronic major depression) in comparison to relatives of episodic depressives. This was largely due to familial aggregation of dysthymia, with relatives of dysthymic probands having an 8.0-fold increase in risk of dysthymia compared to relatives of normals and a 3.6-fold increase in risk of dysthymia compared to the relatives of episodic depressives. In contrast, chronic major depression aggregated in the families of both dysthymic and episodic major depressive probands. These findings of differing patterns of familial aggregation provide striking support for the view that dysthymia represents a condition that is distinct from, although related to, major depression, whether episodic or chronic.

Rates of bipolar disorders were low in all groups of relatives, thus providing no evidence to support the earlier suggestions of Akiskal and Klein of a familial relationship between dysthymia and bipolar disorder. When comorbidity in the probands was controlled for, relatives of the three proband groups had similar rates of all other Axis I disorders as well, except for panic disorder, which was higher in the relatives of dysthymic probands. This unexpected finding also contrasts with the analysis of Goodman et al., who observed no increase in rates of dysthymia in relatives of probands with panic disorder, and may require further study.

Analysis of the personality disorder diagnoses revealed an interesting pattern of associations. Dysthymic probands had significantly higher rates of personality disorders than the episodic depressives (60% versus 18%) or the normal controls, who by definition had no personality disorder diagnosis. When proband comorbidity with personality disorders was controlled for, relatives of dysthymic and episodic major depressive probands compared to relatives of normals had increased risks of any personality disorder; of any Cluster A, B, or C personality disorder, considering each cluster separately; and of most of the individual personality disorders. Relatives of dysthymic and episodic major depressive probands only differed from each other in the finding that relatives of dysthymic probands had an increased risk of passive-aggressive personality disorder. However, when proband comorbidity with personality disorders was not controlled for, relatives of dysthymic probands had significantly higher rates of any personality disorder and any Cluster B disorder compared to relatives of episodic major depressive probands. The data thus appear to suggest that although dysthymia is associated with personality disorders in both probands themselves and their relatives, the association between personality disorders and dysthymia is not a simple one and that episodic depression shares with dysthymia a familial association with personality disorders that is independent of comorbid personality disorders in the probands.

Klein et al. further subdivided the dysthymic probands into subjects with and without a lifetime history of superimposed major depression. Relatives of these two groups of dysthymic probands did not differ on rates of any Axis I or Axis II disorder. Furthermore, when relatives of these two proband groups were compared separately to the relatives of episodic major depressives and normal controls, the relatives of the double depressives resembled those of the pure dysthymic probands much more than they did the relatives of the episodic depressives. Klein et al. suggest that these finding support the view that the underlying pattern of mild chronic depression seen in dysthymia with or without major depression may ultimately be of greater significance than the superimposed episodes of greater symptomatology seen in double depressives.

## *Discussion of Family Studies*

Taken as a whole, the family studies to date provide convincing evidence that dysthymia is both related to major depression and yet distinct from it inasmuch as dysthymia breeds true in families and is associated with a pattern of comorbid diagnoses that differs from that found in probands with major depression alone. The results of Klein's well-designed study of both personality diagnoses and Axis I disorders are not consistent with the view that dysthymia is purely a manifestation of personality disorder. Dysthymia resembles episodic major depression in that both are associated with a wide range of personality disorders in relatives irrespective of proband comorbidity. However, the observation that dysthymic probands themselves, as compared to episodic depressives, have increased comorbidity with personality disorders and that rates of personality disorders are highest in relatives of dysthymics when proband comorbidity is not controlled for suggests that there are some differences as well between episodic depressives and dysthymics in the relationship between personality and mood disorders.

In part, the debates over the nature of chronic depression—whether it is closer to mood disorders or to personality disorders—reflect underlying differing viewpoints of what factors are not only associated with dysthymia but also causally related to it. The aforementioned studies provide little information about the role of potential etiologic factors in dysthymia. Akiskal et al. observed a 60% rate of "developmental object loss" (including parental divorce, death, proband adoption, or living in a foster home or orphanage) in the subset of early-onset chronic depressives with character-spectrum disorder. They also found that these probands frequently described a tempestuous life style in their parents. Akiskal's subaffective dysthymics reported much lower rates of such environmental risk factors. These findings suggest a significant role for environmental causation in a subset of early-onset chronic depressives and potentially a more genetic etiology for another group. While this study has generated hypotheses about the role of environmental risk factors in chronic depression, further research using reliable instruments for diagnosis and for assessment of environmental risk factors will be needed. Direct studies of genetic factors in chronic depression (twin and adoption studies) are also limited by their reliance on diagnostic assessments of questionable relevance and reliability. All have significant methodologic weaknesses as well and rely on current and former diagnostic conceptualizations of chronic depression that may not adequately capture the diagnostic complexities and possible heterogeneity of chronic depressives.

## Twin Studies

Torgersen's (1986) twin study of affective disorders is the only twin or adoption study that uses modern diagnostic criteria for chronic depression. Among 151 index twins with moderately severe and mild affective disorders, 16 monozygotic (MZ) and 19 dizygotic (DZ) twins received a diagnosis of dysthymic disorder. There was a 25% (4/16) concordance rate for any affective disorder among the MZ co-twins of dysthymic probands and a 16% (3/19) concordance rate among the DZ co-twins. Of the 16 MZ co-twins, 3 (19%) had dysthymic disorder and none had major depression whereas 1 of the 19 DZ co-twins (5%) had dysthymic disorder and 2 of 19 (11%) had major depression. MZ co-twins of probands with major depression had higher rates of dysthymic disorder (5/33, or 15%) than DZ co-twins (5/59, or 8%).

These results provide little evidence of important hereditary factors in dysthymic disorder since concordance rates of MZ and DZ twin pairs are low for dysthymic disorder. The 25% concordance rate for any affective illness in MZ co-twins of dysthymic probands most clearly suggests that genetic factors have a limited role in the etiology of this condition. However, Torgersen's study had marked limitations. The sample of dysthymics is small and is not well characterized. Age of onset (early or late) was not specified. Comorbidity with anxiety, substance abuse, and personality disorders was not described. A diagnostic hierarchy was used whereby dysthymic disorder was not diagnosed if major depression was present, a decision that would be expected to decrease the evidence for genetic factors in dysthymic disorder. Furthermore, all diagnoses were made on the basis of nonblind interviews using the Present State Examination (PSE), which Torgersen personally administered to all twins. The PSE is based on the International Classification of Diseases, and although Torgersen asserted that making DSM-III diagnoses on the basis of the PSE (using a computer algorithm) was "easier than expected," the reliability of this diagnostic approach is untested.

Older twin and adoption studies of neurotic depression may also shed some light on the role of genetic factors in chronic depression. Although the concept of neurotic depression differs from dysthymic disorder and dysthymia, there is significant overlap between the categories (Klein et al., 1993). Studies of neurotic depression, therefore, while lacking the more rigorous diagnostic methodologies of more modern studies, are potentially relevant to an understanding of chronic depression.

The Maudsley twin study assessed the presence of anxiety, depressive neuroses, and personality disorders (Slater & Cowie, 1971; Tsuang & Faraone, 1990). Unlike Torgersen's study, diagnoses were made blind to the diagnosis of the co-twin. For probands with neurotic depression, 25% of their MZ co-twins and 24% of their DZ co-twins had a psychiatric diagnosis, but none of the co-twins received a diagnosis of neurotic depression. By contrast, 41% of MZ co-twins but only 4% of DZ co-twins of probands with anxiety neurosis were concordant for the specific diagnosis of anxiety neurosis, and concordance rates for any psychiatric diagnosis were higher. While population base rates would be important to fully interpret the results of this study, the Maudsley study found no genetic effect in depressive neurosis but a substantial one for anxiety neurosis. Again, however, questions about the reliability and validity of the diagnostic assessments in this study limit its power.

Shapiro's (1970) twin study of neurotic depression, like the Maudsley study, concluded that there is little evidence for genetic factors in neurotic depression. The Shapiro study, the only English-language study of neurotic depression to publish case histories of the entire sample, compared concordance rates among MZ and DZ twin pairs in which at least one twin had been hospitalized for nonendogenous depression. Concordance rates for both MZ and DZ twins were low, with little difference between the two groups, suggesting a minimal role for genetic factors in neurotic depression. However, Englund and Klein (1990), in a reanalysis of the Shapiro data in which more reliable diagnostic methodologies and more modern diagnostic criteria were used, found substantially more evidence for genetic factors in neurotic depression. The Englund and Klein analysis is therefore of interest not only because it suggests a more significant role for genetic factors in neurotic depression than other studies have found but also because it suggests that methodologic weaknesses, such as those in Shapiro's study, may explain the failure of other studies to find evidence for genetic factors in neurotic depression.

In order to rediagnose all subjects according to RDC (Spitzer,

Endicott, & Robins, 1978) for major or minor depression and simultaneously to Winokur's (1985) proposed formal diagnostic criteria for neurotic–reactive depression, Englund and Klein used edited versions of Shapiro's case histories from which all references to zygosity had been removed. Diagnostic reliability, determined by using two independent diagnostic raters who were blind to both zygosity and co-twin diagnosis, was good. Among the 16 MZ probands who met both RDC criteria for major or minor depression and Winokur's criteria for neurotic depression, 10 of 16 co-twins met criteria for RDC major or minor depression and 6 of 16 co-twins met criteria for neurotic depression as well. Among the 11 DZ probands, however, only 2 met criteria for RDC major or minor depression and none for neurotic depression. Although this study suffers as well from significant limitations primarily derived from the original sample, including the lack of blind diagnostic case histories by Shapiro, the Englund and Klein reanalysis suggests not only that the Shapiro cases indicate a significantly greater role for genetic factors in neurotic depression than has been found by other investigators but also that methodological weaknesses in other twin studies may have contributed to the lack of evidence of genetic factors in chronic depressions.

## An Adoption Study

The study by Wender et al. (1986) of psychiatric disorders in biologic and adoptive families of Danish adoptees with mood disorders found evidence of a genetic component to the major mood disorders (which included unipolar and bipolar disorder and a category with "uncertain major mood disorder") but failed to find evidence for a substantial genetic effect in neurotic depression. Seventy-one adoptees with a history of hospitalization for mood disorders (unipolar and bipolar disorder, neurotic depression, and "affect reaction"—a Danish diagnosis for individuals with histrionic or impulsive behavior in response to an identifiable stressor) were compared to 75 adoptees with no history of psychiatric hospitalization. Diagnostic information on all probands, adoptive relatives, and biologic relatives was obtained from the national Psychiatric Register (which contains records of psychiatric hospitalizations in Denmark) and from police reports of suicide attempts and completions. No direct interview data were available. Biologic relatives of ill adoptees had significantly higher rates of major mood disorders, unipolar depression, alcohol abuse and dependence, and suicide. Rates of neurotic depression in the biologic relatives of ill and control adoptees, in contrast, were identical (7/387 and 6/344, respectively). This study suffered, however, from a crucial methodologic weakness: Since ill probands were ascertained on the basis of psychiatric hospitalization and assessment of psychopathology in relatives was also based on hospitalization and police records, this study had no power to detect genetic factors in psychiatric disorders that were not severe enough to warrant hospitalization or to lead to a suicide attempt. While many chronic depressives certainly have histories of psychiatric hospitalizations, milder chronic depressions would have escaped analysis in this study. As Englund and Klein's reanalysis of Shapiro's data suggests, evidence for genetic factors in neurotic depression may be overlooked if psychiatric diagnoses are only made on the basis of hospitalization.

## Summary

In summary, while data from family studies of chronic depressives are limited, genetic and environmental studies of families of chronic depressives are even scarcer. Family data provide strong evidence of a relationship between dysthymia and unipolar depression and of the validity of at least the early-onset form of dysthymia as a distinct entity manifesting familial transmission. Less is known about the nature of the familial associations between personality disorders and depression, whether chronic or episodic. Chronic depressives may be a heterogeneous group, but rigorous studies using reliable methodologies have not yet supported the validity of any proposed subcategories. Finally, and perhaps most importantly, the role of specific genetic and environmental factors in chronic depression remains unclear, there being some initial evidence from Akiskal's study for a significant environmental contribution but minimal reliable data on genetic factors. Clarification of these issues will require further study.

## Acknowledgment

This work was supported in part by a Research Fellowship from the DeWitt Wallace/New York Hospital Fund and by Grant No. R01-MH37103 from the National Institute of Mental Health.

## References

Akiskal, H. S., King, D., Rosenthal, T. L., Robinson, D., Scott-Strauss, A. (1981). Chronic depressions: Part 1. Clinical and familial characteristics in 137 probands. *Journal of Affective Disorders, 3*, 297–315.

American Psychiatric Association. (1980). *Diagnostic and statistical manual of mental disorders* (3rd ed.). Washington, DC: Author.

American Psychiatric Association. (1987). *Diagnostic and statistical manual of mental disorders* (3rd ed., rev.). Washington, DC: Author.

American Psychiatric Association. (1994). *Diagnostic and statistical manual of mental disorders* (4th ed.). Washington, DC: Author.

Angst, J., & Wicki, W. (1991). The Zurich Study: XI. Is dysthymia a separate form of depression? Results of the Zurich Cohort Study. *European Archives of Psychiatry and Clinical Neuroscience, 240*, 349–354.

Cloninger, C. R., Reich, T., & Wetzel, R. (1979). Alcoholism and affective disorders: Familial associations and genetic models. In D. W. Goodwin & C. K. Erickson (Eds.), *Alcoholism and affective disorders* (pp. 57–87). New York: Spectrum.

Englund, S. A., & Klein, D. N. (1990). The genetics of neurotic–reactive depression: A reanalysis of Shapiro's (1970) twin study using diagnostic criteria. *Journal of Affective Disorders, 18*, 247–252.

Frances, A. (1980). The DSM-III personality disorders section: A commentary. *American Journal of Psychiatry, 137*, 1050–1054.

Frances, A., & Cooper, A. M. (1981). Descriptive and dynamic psychiatry: A persective on DSM-III. *American Journal of Psychiatry, 138*, 1198–1202.

Friedman, R. A. (1993). Social impairment in dysthymia. *Psychiatric Annals, 23*, 632–637.

Goodman, D. W., Goldstein, R. B., Adams, P. B., Horwath, E., Sobin, C., Wickramaratne, P., & Weissman, M. M. (in press). The relationship between dysthymia and major depression: An analysis of family study data. *Depression*.

Hesselbrock, V., Tennen, H., Stabinau, J., & Hesselbrock, M. (1983). Affective disorder in alcoholism. *International Journal of the Addictions, 18*, 435–444.

Klein, D. N., Clark, D. C., Dansky, L., & Margolis, E. T. (1988). Dysthymia in the offspring of parents with primary unipolar affective disorder. *Journal of Abnormal Psychology, 97*, 265–274.

Klein, D. N., Riso, L. P., & Anderson, R. L. (1993). DSM-III-R Dysthymia: Antecedents and underlying assumptions. In L. J. Chapman, J. P. Chapman, & D. C. Fowles (Eds.), *Progress in experimental personality and psychopathology research* (Vol. 16, pp. 222–253). New York: Springer.

Klein, D. N., Riso, L. P., Donaldson, S. K., Schwartz, J. E., Anderson, R. L., Ouimette, P. C., Lizardi, H., & Aronson, T. A. (1995). *A family study of early-onset dysthymia.* Manuscript submitted for publication.

Klein, D. N., Taylor, E. B., Dickstein, S., & Harding, K. (1988). Primary early-onset dysthymia: Comparison with primary nonbipolar nonchronic major depression on demographic, clinical, familial, personality, and socioenvironmental characteristics and short-term outcome. *Journal of Abnormal Psychology, 97*, 387–398.

Kocsis, J. H., & Frances, A. J. (1987). A critical discussion of DSM-III dysthymic disorder. *American Journal of Psychiatry, 144*, 1534–1542.

Markowitz, J. C., Moran, M. E., Kocsis, J. H., & Frances, A. J. (1992). Prevalence and comorbidity of dysthymic disorder among psychiatric outpatients. *Journal of Affective Disorders, 24*, 63–71.

Robins, E., & Guze, S. B. (1970). Establishment of diagnostic validity in psychiatric illness: Its application to schizophrenia. *American Journal of Psychiatry, 126*, 983–987.

Shapiro, R. W. (1970). A twin study of non-endogenous depression. *Acta Jutland*, 42, 1–179.

Slater, E., & Cowie, V. (1971). *The genetics of mental disorder.* London: Oxford University Press.

Spitzer, R. L., Endicott, J., & Robins, E. (1978). Research Diagnostic Criteria: Rationale and reliability. *Archives of General Psychiatry, 35*, 773–782.

Torgersen, S. (1986). Genetic factors in moderately severe and mild affective disorders. *Archives of General Psychiatry, 43*, 222–226 .

Tsuang, M. T., & Faraone, S. V. (1990). *The genetics of mood disorders.* Baltimore: Johns Hopkins University Press.

Weissman, M. M., Leaf, P. J., Bruce, M. L., Florio, L. (1988). The epidemiology of dysthymia in five communities: Rates, risks, comorbidity, and treatment. *American Journal of Psychiatry, 145*, 815–819.

Weissman, M. M., Merikangas, K. R., John, K., Wickramaratne, P., Prusoff, B. A., & Kidd, K. K. (1986). Family–genetic studies of psychiatric disorders: Developing technologies. *Archives of General Psychiatry, 43*, 1104–1116.

Weissman, M. M., Wickramaratne, P., Adams, P. B., Lish, J. D., Horwath, E., Charney, D., Woods, S. W., Leeman, E., & Frosch, E. (1993). The relationship between panic disorder and major depression: A new family study. *Archives of General Psychiatry, 50*, 767–780.

Weissman, M. M., Wickramaratne, P., Merikangas, K. R., Leckman, J. F., Prusoff, B. A., Caruso, K. A., Kidd, K. K., & Gammon, G. D. (1984). Onset of major depression in early adulthood: Increased familial loading and specificity. *Archives of General Psychiatry, 41*, 1136–1143.

Wender, P. H., Kety, S. S., Rosenthal, D., Schulsinger, F., Ortmann, J., & Lunde, I. (1986). Psychiatric disorders in the biological and adoptive families of adopted individuals with affective disorders. *Archives of General Psychiatry, 43*, 923–929.

Winokur, G. (1985). The validity of neurotic-reactive depression: New data and reappraisal. *Archives of General Psychiatry, 42*, 1116–1122.

CHAPTER EIGHT

# Pharmacotherapy of Dysthymic Disorder

WILMA M. HARRISON
JONATHAN W. STEWART

A recent epidemiologic study, the National Comorbidity Survey, has confirmed earlier reports indicating a high prevalence for dysthymic disorder (Kessler et al., 1994). Despite the high lifetime prevalence of dysthymic disorder and associated morbidity and psychosocial impairment, there has been surprisingly little systematic study of pharmacotherapy or psychotherapy as treatments for this disorder in contrast to major depression. The clinician has few empirically based guidelines for selection of the most promising treatment.

Like other forms of chronic depression, dysthymic disorder has often been unrecognized or underdiagnosed and untreated (Weissman & Klerman, 1977). Even when detected, mild protracted depression has been thought to be a symptom of an underlying character disorder, and a depression best treated with psychotherapy. If medications are tried, the dose and/or duration of treatment is usually inadequate. This may reflect therapeutic nihilism stemming from the perception of chronic depression as a medication-resistant condition or from the assumption that milder depression warrants lower doses.

The classification of dysthymic disorder among the affective disorders in DSM-III stimulated interest in pharmacologic treatments for chronic low-grade depression. Akiskal's (1983) early uncontrolled study of pharmacotherapy response in chronic depression had suggested that some patients have a subsyndromal variant of affective disorder while others who are unresponsive to medication have "characterological depression." Other factors that contributed to the emerging interest in pharmacotherapy of dysthymic disorder included greater awareness of chronic depression as a residual of inadequately treated major depression and the recognition that major depression is typically a chronic or recurrent illness requiring continued treatment (Keller & Shapiro, 1982).

Newer antidepressants with fewer unpleasant side effects of the type likely to lead to discontinuation have been developed during the past decade. The new agents include the selective serotonin reuptake inhibitors (SSRIs), serotonin antagonists, and reversible inhibitors of monoamine oxidase type A. These drugs, with their more tolerable side effect profiles, make it easier to treat patients with chronic depression who may need to take antidepressants for prolonged periods.

With the shift in conceptualization of dysthymic disorder and the advent of new antidepressants, systematic studies of pharmacologic treatment for dysthymic disorder were initiated. Earlier open and uncontrolled studies of pharmacotherapy for minor depressions had suggested that antidepressant medications were effective for many patients (Stewart, Quitkin, & Klein, 1992).

Two recent publications provide comprehensive reviews of open as well as controlled pharmacologic trials in various forms of minor depression and dysthymia (Conte & Karasu, 1992; Howland, 1991). While the studies reviewed provide suggestive evidence of effectiveness in dysthymic disorder, they are not conclusive because of a variety of methodologic flaws, which include brief duration, small and heterogeneous samples, inclusion of patients with concurrent major depression, lack of placebo controls, use of concomitant psychotropic medications, and failure to use a rigorous definition of response (i.e., recovery from dysthymia).

In order to develop recommendations for treatment strategies, we need to know the answers to the following questions: (1) Is there evidence from placebo-controlled clinical trials to substantiate the efficacy of antidepressant treatment of dysthymia with and without concurrent major depression? (2) What is the optimum duration of treatment for dysthymia? (3) Are there differences in treatment response or tolerability favoring a particular class of medication? (4) Do the results of controlled treatment studies provide information about the type of dysthymic patient most likely to respond to medication?

## Literature Review

The following literature review focuses primarily on controlled double-blind studies of patients with disorders defined by DSM-III (American Psychiatric Association, 1980) or DSM-III-R (American Psychiatric Association, 1987) in order to best evaluate the evidence for the efficacy of pharmacotherapy in dysthymic disorder and address the aforementioned four questions. The studies have been grouped according to whether they include patients with a concurrent major depression, that is, patients with double depression (Table 8.1), or exclude them, thus yielding patients with pure dysthymic disorder (Table 8.2). The majority of the studies failed to exclude patients who were in an episode of major depression at the time of study entry, or they required a minimum Hamilton Rating Scale for Depression (HRSD) score for study inclusion that was high enough to make it likely that the patient was experiencing an episode of major depression when baselines were assessed. This makes it difficult to determine whether a responder to medication had merely experienced a remission of the superimposed exacerbation of depression or had actually recovered from the underlying dysthymia. In some trials the description of the study sample suggests that patients suffering from a partially remitted major depressive episode or chronic major depression were included.

*Is there evidence from placebo-controlled trials to substantiate the efficacy of antidepressant therapy in dysthymic disorder with and without comorbid major depression?* The first well-designed placebo-controlled trial in dysthymic disorder, conducted by Kocsis et al. (1988), compared imipramine with placebo in a 6-week study in 76 patients with DSM-III dysthymic disorder of whom 96% met criteria for a current major depression. The average daily peak dose of imipramine was 198 ± 59 mg, and the average plasma drug concentration at steady state was 276 ± 116 ng/ml. The researchers prospectively designated criteria for response that differentiated patients who had full remission (HRSD score < 7) from those who

**TABLE 8.1. Pharmacotherapy of Double Depression**

| Study | Number of patients | Diagnosis/severity | Duration | Drug | Maximum dose | Results |
|---|---|---|---|---|---|---|
| Kocsis et al. (1988) | 76 | DSM-III and HRSD ≥ 14 | 6 weeks | Imipramine vs. placebo | 300 mg | Imipramine > placebo |
| Geisler, Mygind, Knudsen, & Sloth-Nielson (1992) | 67 | DSM-III and HRSD > 15 | 6 weeks | Ritanserin vs. flupenthixol | 10 mg<br>2 mg | Ritanserin = flupenthixol |
| Vallejo, Gasto, & Catalan (1987) | 39 | DSM-III and HRSD > 16 | 6 weeks | Imipramine vs. phenelzine | 250 mg<br>75 mg | Imipramine < phenelzine |
| Reyntjens, Gelders, Hoppenbrouwers, & Bussche (1986) | 57 | DSM-III and moderate symptomatology | 6 weeks | Ritanserin vs. placebo | 20 mg | Ritanserin > placebo |
| Bersani et al. (1991) | 30 | DSM-III and HRSD > 20 | 5 weeks | Ritanserin vs. placebo | 10 mg | Ritanserin > placebo |
| Guelfi, Pichot, & Dreyfus (1989) | 265 | DSM-III and MADRS > 20 and anxiety | 6 weeks | Tianeptine vs. amitriptyline | 50 mg<br>100 mg | Tianeptine = amitriptyline |
| Keller et al. (1995) | 95 | DSM-III-R and HRSD > 18 | 12 weeks | Imipramine vs. sertraline | 300 mg<br>200 mg | Sertraline = imipramine |
| Lecrubier (1994) | 219 | DSM-III-R | 6 weeks | Imipramine vs. amisulpride vs. placebo | 100 mg<br>50 mg | Imipramine > placebo<br>Amisulpride > placebo |

*Note*. Double depression = concurrent major depression and dysthymia.

TABLE 8.2. Pharmacotherapy of Pure Dysthymia

| Study | Number of patients | Diagnosis/severity | Duration | Drug | Maximum dose | Results |
|---|---|---|---|---|---|---|
| Hellerstein, Yanowitch, & Rosenthal (1992) | 32 | DSM-III-R; primary, early onset | 8 weeks | Fluoxetine vs. placebo | 60 mg | Fluoxetine > placebo |
| Versiani (1993)[a] | 315 | DSM-III-R and at least moderate severity | 8 weeks | Moclobemide vs. imipramine vs. placebo | 700 mg<br>250 mg | Moclobemide > placebo<br>Imipramine > placebo |
| Kocsis, Thase, Koran, Halbreich, & Yonkers (1994) | 416 | DSM-III-R; primary, early onset | 12 weeks | Sertraline vs. imipramine vs. placebo | 200 mg<br>300 mg | Sertraline > placebo<br>Imipramine > placebo<br>Sertraline = imipramine |
| Stewart, McGrath, & Quitkin (1989) | 57 | DSM-III and HRSD > 10 | 6 weeks | Imipramine vs. phenelzine vs. placebo | 300 mg<br>90 mg | Imipramine > placebo<br>Phenelzine = placebo<br>Imipramine = phenelzine |
| Stewart, McGrath, & Liebowitz (1985) | 18 | DSM-III and HRSD ≤ 18 | 6 weeks | Desipramine vs. placebo | 300 mg | Desipramine = placebo |
| Bakish et al. (1993) | 50 | DSM-III and HRSD ≥ 13 | 7 weeks | Imipramine vs. ritanserin vs. placebo | 200 mg<br>20 mg | Imipramine > placebo<br>Ritanserin > placebo<br>Imipramine = ritanserin |

*Note.* Pure dysthymia = dysthymia without concurrent major depression.

had clinically significant improvement (defined as HRSD score $< 12$). Fifty-nine percent of imipramine-treated completers and 13% of placebo completers were full or partial responders. When nonresponse rates were recalculated by classifying dropouts as nonresponders, the response rates (45% in the imipramine group and 12% in the placebo group) were lower but remained significantly different. While it is probable that most of the patients in the full remission group had achieved recovery from dysthymic disorder, this was not evaluated.

Stewart, McGrath, and Quitkin (1989) studied 57 patients with DSM-III dysthymic disorder and "atypical depression" (according to Columbia University criteria; Stewart, McGrath, Rabkin, & Quitkin, 1993) without comorbid major depression in a 6-week double-blind study comparing imipramine, phenelzine, and placebo. Response was based on a Clinical Global Impression (CGI) improvement rating of "very much" or "much improved," but patients were not assessed for presence of dysthymic disorder at the end of treatment. Seventy-eight percent of the imipramine group and 58% of the phenelzine group who completed treatment responded, in contrast to 33% of the placebo-treated patients. While there was no statistically significant difference between the two active drugs, only imipramine was superior to placebo ($p < .05$).

In an earlier trial Stewart, McGrath, and Liebowitz (1985) failed to demonstrate a difference between desipramine and placebo. This study, however, included a very small group of dysthymics (only 9 patients per treatment group) and the use of retrospective diagnoses based on an algorithm that converted Research Diagnostic Criteria (RDC) diagnoses into DSM-III categories.

Bersani et al. (1991) compared ritanserin with placebo in a 6-week double-blind trial in patients with DSM-III dysthymic disorder. Seventy-five percent of the ritanserin patients were considered to have a marked or moderate therapeutic response, but only 18% of the placebo-treated patients achieved this degree of response. The ritanserin-treated patients had a significantly greater decrease in HRSD scores than the placebo group. However, the mean posttreatment HRSD score in the ritanserin group was $13.9 \pm 1.3$ (*SE*), which suggests the persistence of residual depression. There was no assessment of the number of patients who continued to meet criteria for dysthymic disorder at the completion of treatment.

Another study, by Reyntjens, Gelders, Hoppenbrouwers, and Bussche (1986), entered 93 patients with DSM-III dysthymic disorder and moderately severe symptoms in a 6-week double-blind placebo-controlled trial of ritanserin. The dropout rate was high (36 of 93), and response criteria were loosely defined. Of the completers, 63% of the ritanserin group were considered to have had an excellent or good therapeutic effect, compared with 41% of the placebo-treated group, a nonsignificant difference.

Lecrubier (1994) reported results of a study comparing imipramine, amisulpride, and placebo in 219 patients with DSM-III-R dysthymia. Amisulpride, an atypical antipsychotic, is a substituted benzamide dopamine blocker with greater specificity for $D_2$ and $D_3$ receptors. This drug is marketed in Europe but not in the United States. Half of these dysthymic patients had concomitant major depression. When response was defined as a 50% or greater reduction in Montgomery–Asberg Depression Rating Scale (MADRS) score, 50% of amisulpride patients were responders, compared with 47% of those treated with imipramine and 29% for placebo.

A study by Vallejo, Gasto, and Catalan (1987) comparing imipramine and phenelzine in a double-blind randomized 6-week trial failed to include a placebo control. The maximum permitted doses were 250 mg for imipramine and 75 mg for phenelzine. The phenelzine-treated group had significantly greater improvement than the imipramine-treated patients on posttreatment ratings, including HRSD scores.

Two other double-blind studies compared two active drugs without a placebo control. Geisler, Mygind, Knudsen, and Sloth-Nielson (1992) studied 67 patients with DSM-III dysthymic disorder and HRSD scores above 15. They were treated with ritanserin or flupenthixol, a neuroleptic drug that is not marketed in the United States, in a multicenter study conducted in general practice settings. There was no difference between the drugs in the proportion of patients judged to be "very much improved" or "much improved" at endpoint. For both treatment groups the mean HRSD scores were significantly reduced from baseline to endpoint. Guelfi, Pichot, and Dreyfus (1989) compared tianeptine, a serotonergic antidepressant that is not marketed in the United States, with the tricyclic amitriptyline in 265 dysthymic patients who had a mixture of depression of moderate severity and anxiety. There were no significant differences between treatments.

Preliminary results of the first phase of a multicenter study comparing sertraline with imipramine in patients with DSM-III-R dysthymia and a concurrent major depression have been presented by Keller et al. (1995) for the first 95 patients who completed the initial 12-week phase. Treatment was initiated at doses of 50 mg for sertraline or imipramine, and the dose was titrated upward to a maximum of 300 mg/day for imipramine and 200 mg/day for sertraline. The overall response rate was 61%. Response was defined as having at least a 50% reduction in HRSD score from baseline and a CGI improvement score of "much improved" or "very much improved" at two consecutive visits at least 2 weeks apart at the end of the study. For both drugs there was a significant improvement in HRSD scores from baseline and the proportion of patients responding was similar for sertraline and imipramine.

There have been five recent controlled trials of antidepressant medication that included patients with DSM-III-R dysthymia without a concurrent major depression (Table 8.2). Hellerstein, Yanowitch, and Rosenthal (1993) compared fluoxetine with placebo in 35 patients who met DSM-III-R criteria for primary early-onset dysthymia but not for a current major depressive episode or major depression in partial remission. Response was defined as a 50% or greater reduction in HRSD score and a score of 1 or 2 ("very much improved" or "much improved") on the improvement scale of the CGI. The mean fluoxetine dose for responders was 35 ± 14 mg/day. Of the 16 fluoxetine-treated patients who completed the trial, 10 responded (62.5%), but only 3 of 16 (18.8%) placebo-treated study completers were considered responders. The authors noted, however, that 6 of the 10 fluoxetine responders still had HRSD scores between 7 and 11 at the end of the study period and that most subjects had some degree of residual symptoms. These included mild depression, reduced energy, and decreased libido.

Bakish et al. (1993) studied 50 patients who met DSM-III criteria for dysthymic disorder but were not in an episode of major depression at the time of study entry. The mean duration of illness was 11 years, and the majority of patients had been in previous treatment with psychotherapy (as had Hellerstein's patients). Both imipramine and ritanserin were found to be superior to placebo, but a statistically significant difference between treatments was not demonstrated until the 6th week of the study. There were no significant differences between the two active drugs.

Neither of these studies in "pure dysthymia" included systematic assessment of whether treatment responders continued to meet the diagnostic criteria for dysthymia. This is an important omission, characteristic of most of the dysthymia studies reviewed. The use of arbitrary cutoff scores on rating scales in order to determine treatment response fails to provide definitive evidence for remission of the dysthymia. It is possible for a patient to have a low final score on the HRSD or a 50% reduction in HRSD score from a baseline of approximately 18, and thus be considered much improved, but still meet criteria for dysthymia. This is especially relevant if the patient entered the study during a period of exacerbation of low-grade chronic depression.

In contrast, Versiani (1993) reported results of an 8-week double-blind placebo-controlled multicenter comparison of moclobemide (mean dose 680 mg) and imipramine (mean dose 220 mg) in which recovery was defined as no longer meeting criteria for dysthymia. Moclobemide is a reversible inhibitor of monoamine oxidase type A that is not marketed in the United States. Two-thirds of the patients in the study sample had pure dysthymia, and one-third had double depression. In this study, response was also presented using CGI improvement ratings. Both active drugs were superior to placebo in pure dysthymia and in double depression, but response rates varied considerably depending on the criteria used. In the pure dysthymia group the proportion of patients no longer meeting DSM-III-R criteria for dysthymia after treatment were as follows: 54% of those receiving moclobemide, 49% of those on imipramine, and 24% of those given placebo. When response was defined as being "much improved" or "very much improved" on the CGI scale, 75% of patients on moclobemide were responders, as were 73% of the patients treated with imipramine; only 26% of the placebo-treated patients were considered responders using this criterion.

Similar rates of remission from pure dysthymia were reported by Marin, Kocsis, Frances, and Parides (1994) in an open study of desipramine treatment of dysthymia patients with and without concurrent major depression. Patients with DSM-III-R dysthymia and scores of more than 10 on the 24-item HRSD (HRSD-24) were included in this study. Desipramine was titrated to 200 mg/day by the end of the 2nd week of treatment and increased to doses above that level, as tolerated, in patients who failed to respond to 200 mg. Desipramine levels were monitored. In this study approximately half of the pure dysthymics achieved complete remission, defined as a 50% reduction in HRSD score from baseline and a final HRSD score of less than 7.

Results of a large placebo-controlled multicenter study comparing imipramine and sertraline in 416 patients with early-onset primary dysthymia without concurrent major depression were presented recently by Kocsis, Thase, Koran, Halbreich, and Yonkers (1994). Inclusion in this study required chronicity of depressive symptoms (a minimum duration of 5 years) but permitted inclusion of patients with a mild degree of severity of depressive illness. The mean baseline 17-item HRSD score in these patients was less than 13, which is considerably lower than the baseline HRSD reported for all previous trials. Both sertraline and imipramine were significantly more effective than placebo, with similar efficacy for the two active treatments. However, of the patient discontinuations because of side effects, only 25% were sertraline-treated patients, compared with 51% for imipramine-treated patients. Imipramine was associated with significantly more side effects than sertraline. Similarly, Bakish et al. (1993) reported better tolerability of a serotonergic antidepressant than of imipramine. This is of clinical relevance since patients with milder levels of depression may be less likely to tolerate tricyclic-related side effects, particularly when prolonged periods of treatment are necessary.

Although many of these controlled studies have methodologic flaws, they provide substantial evidence for the efficacy of pharmacotherapy in the treatment of dysthymia with and without comorbid major depression. Tricyclic antidepressants, monoamine oxidase inhibitors, and serotonergic antidepressants all appear to be effective treatments. The considerable variability of rates of response across studies probably reflects the differences in the criteria used to define treatment response and/or sampling variation. In general, when posttreatment changes in HRSD scores or global clinical ratings were used to assess outcome, response rates were similar to those reported in studies of major depression. Lower response rates were consistently reported when response was defined as no longer meeting the diagnostic criteria for dysthymia. This may also be related to the brief duration of most of the treatment studies. Some dysthymia symptoms may take longer to fully improve than the 5- to 6-week study periods provided. Finally, none of the studies assessed the rate of response to a second antidepressant drug for dysthymia patients who failed on the first medication.

*What is the optimum duration of treatment?* Results of the acute treatment studies suggest short-term effectiveness of antidepressant medications for patients with dysthymia, but the studies typically included treatment periods of only 5 to 8 weeks (with the exception of one 12-week trial). These studies provide no assessment of the persistence of the antidepressant effect, and there are few follow-up or long-term studies.

A naturalistic follow-up of 25 out of 39 (64%) patients who had participated in a 6-week double-blind placebo-controlled imipramine study was conducted 1 year or more after the patients had completed the imipramine study (Kocsis, Sutton, & Frances, 1991). A Longitudinal Interval Follow-Up Evaluation (LIFE; Keller & Shapiro, 1982) and other ratings assessed the course and severity of dysthymia, major depression, and other Axis I disorders, as well as the level of social/vocational functioning and the history of treatment during the poststudy period. Interviews were conducted by a psychiatrist who had no knowledge of the original treatment outcome. Imipramine responders demonstrated a better outcome at follow-up than did nonresponders and noncompleters. Eight of the nine responders who participated in the follow-up study remained recovered. Five of these patients were still taking a tricyclic antidepressant. The other three remained well without medication. In contrast, only two of the nine nonresponders were recovered at follow-up, although the majority had subsequently tried at least one other antidepressant. Of the two nonresponders who had recovered at follow-up, one had responded to continued imipramine and psychotherapy and the other was taking phenelzine. Treatment failure was associated with serious consequences. Three treatment failures (one noncompleter and two nonresponders) were hospitalized during the poststudy period, with two of these patients having made suicide attempts.

In an open study with a 2-month follow-up, patients who met DSM-III-R criteria for dysthymia without comorbid major depression were randomly assigned to 3 months of treatment with either fluoxetine, 20 to 60 mg, or trazodone, 50 to 350 mg (Rosenthal, Hemlock, & Hellerstein, 1992). Patients who were unable to tolerate a 12-week trial of the first medication were crossed over to the alternate treatment. Response was defined as a 50% or greater reduction in HRSD score and a rating of "very much improved" or "much improved" on the CGI improvement scale. Eight of 11 patients who completed fluoxetine trials were considered responders (72%), as were four of the six trazodone completers (66.7%). However, when these patients were followed for an additional 2-month period during which they continued on the same medication, only four of the fluoxetine responders and three trazodone responders sustained the therapeutic response, yielding response rates of 36.4% and 50%, respectively. There are several possible explanations for these results. The initial group of responders may have included patients with a nonspecific response, suggesting that the actual antidepressant response rate in dysthymic patients may be closer to 50% rather than the higher rate of response reported in short-term uncontrolled trials. Alternatively, these results may represent failure to maintain a persistent response. Because of the pattern of waxing and waning symptom severity and the chronicity of dysthymia, there is a need for additional controlled studies of longer duration.

The first controlled maintenance treatment study of dysthymia is currently in progress (Kocsis, in press). This trial has utilized a double-blind placebo discontinuation design. The acute treatment phase consisted of 10 weeks of open desipramine treatment. Responders received an additional 4 months of open continuation treatment with desipramine. After the 6 months of open treatment, responders entered a double-blind maintenance treatment phase in which they were randomly assigned to either desipramine or placebo for an additional 2-year period. Of the 105 patients who entered the acute treatment study, approximately 60% had concurrent major depression (double depression) and the remainder had pure dysthymia. Patients were classified as full or partial responders on completion of the acute treatment phase. For full response the criterion was an HRSD-24 score of 7 or less for at least 4 weeks and for partial response a score of 12 or less for at least 4 weeks. Thirty-one of 99 patients (31%) who completed the acute treatment phase were considered full responders, and 17 of 99 (17%) were partial responders, for a total response rate in the open acute treatment study of almost 50%. In the maintenance phase of the study, which is ongoing, a significantly higher relapse rate is being seen in patients randomized to placebo discontinuation. Of the 38 patients who entered the maintenance phase of the study, 65% randomized to placebo relapsed, but only one of the 20 patients who continued on desipramine relapsed. Relapse was defined as an HRSD-24 score of more than 12 on at least three successive occasions over a 4-week period and a GAF (Global Assessment of Functioning) score of 60 or less or an urgent need for hospitalization or change of treatment for depression. Most of the relapses occurred in the first 3 to 4 months of the maintenance phase.

The only other controlled long-term trial in dysthymia, a small pilot study (Harrison, Rabkin, & Stewart, 1986), also used the double-blind placebo discontinuation design. In this study 12 patients who met DSM-III criteria for dysthymic disorder and had responded to phenelzine during a 6-week trial were randomly assigned to continue on phenelzine for an additional 6-month period or switch to placebo. Fifty-eight percent of the patients had comorbid major depression. All seven of the patients who discontinued to placebo relapsed whereas only one of the five patients who continued on phenelzine did so. Most of the relapses occurred early, during the first few weeks after discontinuation of the active medication.

The results of these studies indicate that most dysthymic patients require continued treatment for periods of at least 6 to 12 months (and probably considerably longer). Controlled studies are needed to assess predictors of relapse and to determine whether medication can be discontinued successfully after longer periods of maintenance antidepressant treatment.

*Which dysthymic patients benefit from medication?* Some dysthymic patients appear to be responsive to antidepressant medication while others do not derive benefit. This suggests that the diagnostic criteria for DSM-III and DSM-III-R identify a heterogeneous group of patients. Most of the published studies of dysthymia did not assess demographic or diagnostic predictors of response, or they failed to identify predictors of treatment outcome. However, Hellerstein et al. (1993) found that a significantly greater number of their fluoxetine responders had first-degree relatives with a mood disorder compared with responders to placebo. Over a decade ago Akiskal (1983) proposed that dysthymics could be divided into "subaffective" and "characterological" subtypes, with the former group having family histories of mood disorders and medication responsivity.

There is some evidence that pharmacotherapy is effective in dysthymic patients with "atypical depression," that is, with reversed vegetative symptoms, lethargy, and pathological rejection sensitivity (Stewart et al., 1989). Comparison of treatment response in a variety of diagnostic subgroups, including atypical depression, and with comorbid anxiety disorders is of interest but will require placebo controls and larger samples than were included in most of the early studies.

A recent study demonstrating a high rate of comorbidity of personality disorders and dysthymia (Markowitz, 1992) has renewed interest in the relationship between dysthymic disorder and personality disorders and the effect of comorbid Axis II disorders on antidepressant treatment outcome in dysthymia. Of equal interest is whether pharmacotherapy of dysthymic disorder improves treatment outcome for a comorbid personality disorder. Future studies of antidepressant treatment of dysthymic disorder should include assessments of personality traits and disorders before and after short-term treatment and at intervals during continuation treatment and follow-up.

There has been little study of the use of biological measures as predictors of treatment response in dysthymia. A review of biological studies in dysthymia included studies of sleep, neuroendocrine measures, and neurotransmitter function. In general, the results were inconclusive as a result of methodological problems (Howland & Thase, 1991). However, Ravindran et al. (1993) recently reported preliminary results of an ongoing evaluation of serotonergic function in patients with DSM-III-R primary early-onset dysthymia. Prior to initiating treatment with an SSRI (fluoxetine or sertraline), they assessed the following: 24-hour urinary excretion of the serotonin metabolite 5-hydroxyindoleacetic acid (5-HIAA), platelet serotonin uptake, and paroxetine binding in platelets. Treatment responders had significantly lower pretreatment urinary excretion of 5-HIAA than nonresponders. Although the dysthymic patients had reduced platelet serotonin uptake compared with control subjects, lower platelet serotonin uptake did not predict treatment response.

*Are there differences between specific antidepressant medications or classes of drugs in efficacy or tolerability when used to treat dysthymia?* There is insufficient evidence from published controlled trials to answer this question. It is not appropriate to make comparisons of treatments across trials because of differences in study methodology and subject selection. Similar rates of discontinuations for adverse events were generally reported for the drugs studied, and the specific types of side effects reflected the pharmacologic properties of the drugs. There was some evidence suggesting better toleration of serotonergic antidepressants than tricyclics. Since most of the studies were of brief duration, differences between drugs in long-term tolerability could not be evaluated. Controlled studies with adequate sample sizes are needed to assess the comparative efficacy and tolerability of antidepressant medications of different types in the treatment of dysthymic disorder.

In summary, there are placebo-controlled studies that provide convincing evidence for the efficacy of antidepressants in pure dysthymia and double depression. However, most of the studies have important limitations that interfere with our ability to generalize from their results to clinical practice. In general, the duration of treatment was brief, and most patients had either concurrent major depression or an exacerbation of depressive symptom severity at the time of study entry. This was apparent on review of study entry criteria, which usually required either a minimum HRSD score or the presence of moderate or greater severity of illness for inclusion, and from inspection of mean baseline HRSD scores. The mildly depressed dysthymic patients encountered in general psychiatry or primary care offices were generally not studied. On the other hand, the exclusion of patients with comorbid anxiety, substance abuse, and personality disorder in most of the trials makes it difficult to apply the results to the typical dysthymic patient seen in specialty psychiatric clinics or hospital units.

## Treatment Strategies

There is sufficient evidence from existing studies to warrant the recommendation that patients with dysthymic disorder be given a trial of antidepressant medication. Considering the findings indicating that patients with mild forms of depression have substantial morbidity and disability and that dysthymia may be a risk factor for major depression (Kovacs, Feinberg, & Crouse-Novak, 1984), it is preferable to err on the side of aggressive treatment. The only way to determine whether a dysthymic patient will respond to antidepressant medication is to treat the patient.

Before pharmacotherapy for a patient with long-standing mild depression is begun, a comprehensive evaluation is advisable. This should include a complete medical and psychiatric history. It is important to inquire whether the patient is taking prescribed or over-the-counter medications that could be associated with depression. Some patients with chronic depression have been taking benzodiazepines, sedatives, or opiate analgesics for years. Abuse of sedatives may be overlooked when they are taken as components of headache or pain preparations (e.g., barbiturates in Fiorinal). The possibility of other substance abuse should also be assessed. Hormonal preparations prescribed for contraception or as menopausal replacement therapy should also be considered as a possible contributory factor.

Sequential trials of at least two antidepressants of different classes, given in adequate doses for an appropriate duration, should be provided before abandoning pharmacologic treatment. Despite the fact that it has been the practice to use lower doses of medication for treatment of dysthymia than for major depression, there is no evidence to support this approach. On the basis of our own clinical experience we advocate vigorous trials (i.e., maximum tolerated doses) of antidepressant medication in the treatment of dysthymic disorder.

Achieving an adequate dosage in dysthymic patients can be a therapeutic challenge for the clinician. Some patients with mild dysthymia are less willing to tolerate side effects than those with severe major depression. In order to minimize noncompliance or premature termination, it is important to educate patients about possible side effects and reassure them of the likelihood that most will diminish with time. Compliance may also be improved if patients are informed that improvement often takes several weeks and that a full response may require months of treatment. They should be prepared for the possibility that several trials might be necessary before an effective medication is found. It is helpful to initiate treatment with the lowest dose possible and titrate up slowly. Once an effective dose has been determined, it should be maintained during continuation therapy.

In the event of failure to respond to medications, plasma drug concentrations may be assessed. This is particularly advisable in the case of drugs with established concentration–response relationships, such as certain tricyclics, because of the wide intersubject variability in blood levels. In compliant patients with low tricyclic plasma concentrations the dose should be increased and plasma concentrations monitored. Education and counseling should be provided for noncompliant patients in order to achieve an adequate trial of pharmacotherapy. Perhaps the greatest challenge to the clinician treating dysthymic disorder is convincing patients to give medication a fair trial. Many patients with dysthymic disorder have suffered for most of their lives with their illness. They may be pessimistic and highly skeptical about the utility of pharmacotherapy. Alternatively, they may be fearful that if they do obtain a positive response they will have to take medication for the rest of their lives. Education for patients and their families may alleviate some concerns about dependence on drugs and the stigma associated with the need for continued medication.

The following treatment recommendations are based on the clinical experience of the authors, who recognize that alternative strategies may have equal merit. In our opinion, the choice of initial therapy depends on several clinical considerations, including prior treatment history, family history of antidepressant treatment response, medical status, and predominant symptom pattern. Sedating antidepressants may be helpful for patients with insomnia. SSRIs and monoamine oxidase inhibitors (MAOIs) may preferentially target lethargy and atypical vegetative symptoms. We prefer to begin pharmacotherapy for most patients with an SSRI (20 mg of fluoxetine or 50 mg of sertraline). There are no reports of studies of paroxetine in dysthymia, but it is another choice within this class. The initial dose of the SSRI should be maintained for several weeks in order to assess response. If the dysthymia has not fully remitted and there are no dose-limiting side effects, the dose should be increased at intervals of at least 1 week to the maximum recommended dose.

The SSRIs produce less of the anticholinergic and sedating side effects of tricyclics that patients may find particularly annoying during long-term treatment. In addition, SSRIs are less likely to cause unwanted weight gain. This is particularly important in long-term treatment of women, because weight gain can result in premature discontinuation of medication. SSRIs also have the advantage of a lower risk of fatality in the event of an overdose.

The most common side effects of the SSRIs as a group include gastrointestinal symptoms, insomnia, nervousness, sweating, tremor, dizziness, and somnolence. These tend to be relatively mild and are often time limited. Patients who develop insomnia or anxiety can usually be managed with lower doses, slower titration, or addition of benzodiazepines until tolerance to the side effect develops. Sexual dysfunction is not uncommon with antidepressant medications and can interfere with compliance (Herman, Brotman, & Pollack, 1990). Patients should be asked about sexual side effects. It is important to provide education and reassurance that these side effects are not permanent. Attempts should be made to reduce sexual dysfunction by lowering dosage (in some cases there will be a spontaneous improvement in sexual side effects even with continued treatment). If sexual dysfunction persists and is unacceptable, attempts can be made to counteract this effect. Anecdotal reports suggest that cyproheptadine, bethanechol, yohimbine, or amantadine may be useful in alleviating sexual dysfunction caused by antidepressants, but there have been no controlled studies.

For patients who fail to respond to an SSRI we usually try a tricyclic antidepressant. Both imipramine and desipramine have been shown to be effective in dysthymia (Kocsis et al., 1988; Marin et al., 1994). It is preferable to begin with a low dose and titrate up gradually, as tolerated, to a maximum dose of 300 mg of imipramine or desipramine. If patients have recently discontinued fluoxetine, it is prudent to begin a tricyclic with low doses and titrate up more slowly. Persisting plasma levels of fluoxetine and norfluoxetine may inhibit the cytochrome p450 IID6 isoenzyme that metabolizes tricyclics and can result in elevated plasma tricyclic levels. This is less likely to occur with sertraline (Preskorn et al., 1994). As with the SSRIs, an adequate duration of treatment with a tricyclic is necessary in order to assess response; this should not be less than 6 weeks, and it may take longer to achieve a full therapeutic effect. In cases of partial response after an adequate trial, further dose increases and augmentation strategies may be considered.

There are no controlled trials of augmentation strategies in dysthymia. However, if we accept the premise that there may be a similar underlying pathophysiology for major depression and dysthymic disorder, it is not unreasonable to assume that potentiation of antidepressants with lithium, stimulants, or thyroid hormone may occur and that the use of combinations of SSRIs and tricyclics may be effective in dysthymic patients who have failed monotherapy.

Some clinicians would select bupropion or trazodone for patients who fail to respond to SSRIs and tricyclics. Our preference is to try a trial of an MAOI. Of the older, nonselective MAOIs, phenelzine has been studied in dysthymics and may be particularly beneficial for patients with atypical reversed vegetative symptoms. We have also found tranylcypromine and isocarboxazid to be effective. Although there are no published studies of bupropion treatment of dysthymia, anecdotal reports suggest that it is effective for some patients (Zisook, 1992) and is well tolerated.

Combined treatment (medication and psychotherapy) should be considered when there has been a partial response to an adequate trial of pharmacotherapy alone and there are continuing psychosocial stressors or chronic interpersonal problems.

## Conclusion

Evidence from controlled trials suggests that antidepressant medication is effective for a substantial subset of the heterogeneous group of patients who meet DSM-III-R criteria for dysthymia. The distress of these patients, the chronicity of their illness, and the associated functional impairment warrant an aggressive approach to pharmacotherapy. Sequential trials of another class of antidepressant medication administered in recommended full dosage for an adequate duration should be provided for those who fail to respond to the first medication. Further controlled studies to assess the benefits of combined treatment strategies and to compare the effects of pharmacotherapy and psychotherapy in dysthymia should be conducted. Long-term controlled studies are also needed to demonstrate continued efficacy and tolerability and to assess the optimum duration of treatment for this chronic disorder.

## Acknowledgment

This chapter is adapted from Harrison and Stewart (1993). Copyright 1993 by Slack, Inc. Adapted by permission.

## References

Akiskal, H. S. (1983). Dysthymic disorder: Psychopathology of proposed chronic depressive subtypes. *American Journal of Psychiatry, 140,* 11–20.

American Psychiatric Association. (1980). *Diagnostic and statistical manual of mental disorders* (3rd ed.). Washington, DC: Author.

American Psychiatric Association. (1987). *Diagnostic and statistical manual of mental disorders* (3rd ed., rev.). Washington, DC: Author.

Bakish, D., Lapierre, Y. D., Weinstein, R., Klein, J., Wiens, A., Jones, B., Horn, E., Browne, M., Bourget, O., & Blanchard, A. (1993). Ritanserin, imipramine and placebo in the treatment of dysthymic disorder. *Journal of Clinical Psychopharmacology, 13,* 409–414.

Bersani, G., Pozzi, F., Marini, S., Grispini, A., Pasini, A., & Ciani, N. (1991). 5-$HT_2$ receptor antagonism in dysthymia disorder: A double-blind placebo-controlled study with ritanserin. *Acta Psychiatrica Scandinavica, 83,* 244–248.

Conte, H. R., & Karasu, T. B. (1992). A review of treatment studies of minor depression: 1980–1991. *American Journal of Psychotherapy, 1,* 58–74.

Geisler, A., Mygind, O., Knudsen, R., & Sloth-Nielson, M. (1992). Ritanserin and flupenthixol in dysthymic disorder: A controlled double-blind study in general practice. *Nordic Journal of Psychiatry, 46,* 237–243.

Guelfi, J. D., Pichot, P., & Dreyfus, J. F. (1989). Efficacy of tianeptine in anxious depressed patients. *Neuropsychobiology, 22,* 41–48.

Harrison, W., Rabkin, J., & Stewart, J. W. (1986). Phenelzine for chronic depression: A study of continuation treatment. *Journal of Clinical Psychiatry, 47,* 346–349.

Harrison, W., & Stewart, J. W. (1993). Pharmacotherapy of dysthymia. *Psychiatric Annals, 23,* 638–648.

Hellerstein, D., Yanowitch, P., & Rosenthal, J. (1993). A randomized double-blind study of fluoxetine versus placebo in treatment of dysthymia. *American Journal of Psychiatry, 150,* 1169–1175.

Herman, J. B., Brotman, A. W., & Pollack, M. H. (1990). Fluoxetine-induced sexual dysfunction. *Journal of Clinical Psychiatry, 51,* 25–27.

Howland, R. H. (1991). Pharmacotherapy of dysthymia: A review. *Journal of Clinical Psychopharmacology, 11*, 83–92.

Howland, R. H., & Thase, M. E. (1991). Biological studies of dysthymia. *Biological Psychiatry, 30*, 283–304.

Keller, M. B., Harrison, W., Fawcett, J. A., Gelenberg, A., Hirschfeld, R. M., Klein, D., Kocsis, J., McCullough, J. P., Rush, A. J., Schatzberg, A., & Thase, M. (1995). Treatment of chronic depression with sertraline or imipramine: Preliminary blinded response rates. *Psychopharmacology Bulletin, 31*.

Keller, M. B., & Shapiro, R. W. (1982). "Double depression": Superimposition of acute depressive episodes on chronic depressive disorders. *American Journal of Psychiatry, 139*, 438–442.

Kessler, R. C., McGonagle, K. A., Zhao, S., Nelson, C. B, Hughes, M., Eshleman, S., Wittchen, H. U., & Kendler, K. S. (1994). Lifetime and 12-month prevalence of DSM-III-R psychiatric disorders in the United States: Results from the National Comorbidity Survey. *Archives of General Psychiatry, 51*, 8–19.

Kocsis, J. H. (in press). Chronic depression: Pharmacotherapy studies. In H. S. Akiskal (Ed.), *Chronic depressions and their treatment*. New York: Guilford Press.

Kocsis, J. H., Frances, A. J., Voss, C. B., Mann, J. J., Mason, B. J., & Sweeney, J. (1988). Imipramine treatment for chronic depression. *Archives of General Psychiatry, 45*, 253–257.

Kocsis, J. H., Sutton, B. M., & Frances, A. J. (1991). Long-term follow-up of chronic depression treated with imipramine. *Journal of Clinical Psychiatry, 52*, 56–59.

Kocsis, J. H., Thase, M., Koran, L., Halbreich, U., & Yonkers, K. (1994). Pharmacotherapy of pure dysthymia: Sertraline vs. imipramine and placebo. *European Neuropsychopharmacology, 4*, 204.

Kovacs, M., Feinberg, T. L., & Crouse-Novak, M. (1984). Depressive disorders in childhood: I. A longitudinal prospective study of characteristics and recovery. *Archives of General Psychiatry, 41*, 229–237.

Lecrubier, Y. (1994). The treatment of dysthymics with a dopaminergic presynaptic blocker. *Neuropsychopharmacology, 10*(3S), 302.

Marin, D. B., Kocsis, J. H., Frances, A. J., & Parides, M. (1994). Desipramine for the treatment of "pure" dysthymia versus "double" depression. *American Journal of Psychiatry, 151*, 1079–1080.

Markowitz, J. (1992). Prevalence and comorbidity of dysthymic disorder among psychiatric outpatients. *Journal of Affective Disorders, 24*, 63–71.

Preskorn, S. H., Alderman, J., Chung, M., Harrison, W., Harris, S., & Messig, M. (1994). Pharmacokinetics of desipramine coadministered with sertraline or fluoxetine. *Journal of Clinical Psychopharmacology, 14*, 90–98.

Ravindran, A. V., Chydzik, J., Bialik, R. J., Bakish, O., Hrdina, P. D., & Lapierre, Y. D. (1993, May). *Serotonin in primary dysthymia.* Paper presented at the annual meeting of the American Psychiatric Association, San Francisco.

Reyntjens, A., Gelders, Y. G., Hoppenbrouwers, M. J., & Bussche, G. V. (1986). Thymosthenic effects of ritanserin (R 55667), a centrally acting serotonin-$S_2$ receptor blocker. *Drug Development Research, 8*, 205–211.

Rosenthal, J., Hemlock, C., & Hellerstein, D. (1992). A preliminary study of serotonergic antidepressants in treatment of dysthymia. *Progress in Neuropsychopharmacology and Biological Psychiatry, 16*, 933–941.

Stewart, J. W., McGrath, P. J., & Liebowitz, M. R. (1985). Treatment outcome validation of DSM-III depressive subtypes: Clinical usefulness in outpatients with mild to moderate depression. *Archives of General Psychiatry, 42*, 1148–1153.

Stewart, J. W., McGrath, P. J., & Quitkin, F. M. (1989). Relevance of DSM-III depressive subtype and chronicity to antidepressant efficacy in atypical depression. *Archives of General Psychiatry, 46*, 1080–1087.

Stewart, J. W., McGrath, P. J., Rabkin, J. G., & Quitkin, F. M. (1993). Atypical depression: A valid clinical entity? *Psychiatric Clinics of North America, 16*, 479–495.

Stewart, J. W., Quitkin, F. M., & Klein, D. F. (1992). The pharmacotherapy of minor depression. *American Journal of Psychotherapy, 1*, 23–36.

Vallejo, J., Gasto, C., & Catalan, R. (1987). Double-blind study of imipramine versus phenelzine in melancholic and dysthymic disorders. *British Journal of Psychiatry, 151*, 639–651.

Versiani, M. (1993). Pharmacotherapy of dysthymia: A controlled study with imipramine, moclobemide or placebo. *Neuropsychopharmacology, 10*(3S), 298.

Weissman, M., & Klerman, G. (1977). The chronic depressive in the community: Unrecognized and poorly treated. *Comprehensive Psychiatry, 18*, 523–532.

Zisook, S. (1992). Treatment of dysthymia and atypical depression. *Journal of Clinical Psychiatry, 10*, 15–23.

CHAPTER NINE

# Psychotherapy of Dysthymic Disorder

JOHN C. MARKOWITZ

In an era of sweeping psychopharmacological advances and fading psychotherapeutic reimbursement, the reader may wonder why a chapter should be devoted to the psychotherapy of dysthymic disorder. Has not psychotherapy been rendered superfluous with the advent of fluoxetine? This question reflects a historical turnabout, since until fairly recently psychotherapy was considered to be the treatment of choice for dysthymic patients.

Chronic depression has historically been considered a temperamental or character disorder, that is, depressive personality (Kocsis & Frances, 1987). For most of this century its preferred treatment was felt to be psychotherapy, in which it was generally considered to have a poor prognosis (Akiskal et al., 1980). DSM-III (American Psychiatric Association, 1980) identified chronic depression as dysthymic disorder, an affective syndrome rather than a personality disorder. Successful randomized trials of antidepressant pharmacotherapy for dysthymic disorder followed this nosologic shift (Harrison & Stewart, 1993; Howland, 1991; Kocsis, Frances, Voss, Mann, et al., 1988; Stewart et al., 1988). Since comparable psychotherapeutic outcome trials for dysthymic disorder do not exist, medication should for now be considered its de facto treatment of choice.

In 1984 Weissman and Akiskal proposed research on psychotherapeutic approaches to dysthymic disorder. Noting that only "indirect" evidence existed for psychotherapeutic efficacy in chronic depression, they proposed research on the efficacy of short-term therapies–interpersonal, cognitive, or behavioral–either alone or in combination with medication. Since then, our understanding of dysthymic disorder has greatly improved. DSM-III-R (American Psychiatric Association, 1987) and DSM-IV (American Psychiatric Association, 1994) have sharpened the diagnostic precision of dysthymic disorder. We better understand its high prevalence (Kessler et al., 1994; Weissman, Leaf, Bruce, & Florio, 1988), morbidity (Wells, Burnam, Rogers, Hays, & Camp, 1992; Wells et al., 1989), and comorbidity (see Chapter 3, this volume; Markowitz, Moran, Kocsis, & Frances, 1992; Weissman et al., 1988). Dysthymic disorder now appears not to be a "subsyndromal" disorder, as DSM-III suggested, but a major public health problem. Indeed, the effect of dysthymic disorder on quality of life and functioning has been shown to outweigh that of major depression (Wells et al., 1992), although the latter receives far more research attention.

Clinicians are becoming increasingly aware of controlled clinical trials demonstrating the efficacy of antidepressant medication for many dysthymic patients (Harrison & Stewart, 1993; Howland, 1991; Kocsis, Frances, Voss, & Mann, 1988; Stewart et al., 1988). Randomized clinical trials have also shown the efficacy of time-limited manualized psychotherapies for acute major depression (Beck, Rush, Shaw, & Emery, 1979; Elkin et al., 1989; Klerman, Weissman, Rounsaville, & Chevron, 1984) and for other Axis I disorders. There have been few controlled psychotherapy trials for dysthymia. Compared to other areas of research on dysthymic disorder, psychotherapy has received little attention. Yet dysthymic patients are known to make frequent use of mental health services (Weissman et al., 1988), and it is generally assumed that they account for significant proportions of many, if not most, psychotherapeutic practices.

## Rationale for Antidysthymic Psychotherapy

Since medication can often effectively treat dysthymic disorder, what is the rationale for antidysthymic psychotherapy? Roughly half of dysthymic patients do not respond to antidepressant medication. Others cannot tolerate the side effects, develop hypomania (Akiskal, 1981), or simply refuse medication. Pregnancy and other medical conditions may be relative contraindications to medication. The 3% of American adults who have dysthymic disorder make frequent use of mental health services (Kessler et al., 1994; Weissman et al., 1988), many of them visiting nonpsychiatrists, who (at least at this juncture) cannot prescribe medication. Thus, despite the ascendancy of antidepressant medication as standard treatment for this condition, antidysthymic psychotherapy remains potentially important. Limitations in the efficacy of antidepressant medication, as well as the treatment preference of patients and therapists, argue for the development of effective psychotherapeutic interventions. Dysthymic disorder also offers an interesting target for research on psychotherapeutic efficacy because of its low placebo response rate (Kocsis, Frances, Voss, Mann, et al., 1988).

This chapter reviews recent outcome research on dysthymic disorder with psychotherapy alone or with psychotherapy in combination with antidepressant medication. The literature was searched by using a computerized database and the key words *dysthymia*, *dysthymic disorder*, *chronic depression*, and *psychotherapy* in Excerpta Medica: Psychiatry (Database on CD-ROM, SilverPlatter Version 3.11, Amsterdam: Elsevier Science Publishers, 1980–1993). All studies reporting psychotherapy treatment outcome for dysthymic patients were included except studies of late-life chronic major depression. In reviewing this literature, one should be mindful of distinctions between pure dysthymic disorder and double depression (i.e., major depression superimposed on dysthymic disorder), early- versus late-onset dysthymic disorder, full versus partial remission, and treatment with psychotherapy alone versus psychotherapy in combination with psychopharmacology (Kocsis & Frances, 1987).

I believe that "pure" dysthymic disorder and double depression (Keller, Lavori, Endicott, Coryell, & Klerman, 1983), which differ (in DSM-III, DSM-III-R, and DSM-IV) in number of symptoms while sharing insidious onset and chronicity, are more alike than different. Although Weissman and Akiskal have argued that late-onset chronic depression—essentially unresolved acute depression—might have a better prognosis than early-onset dysthymic disorder, most studies have addressed the latter. (This review ignores the former syndrome, now separately classified in DSM-IV as chronic major depression.)

## Psychotherapy Studies

Akiskal (1980) asserted that chronic depression responds poorly to pharmacotherapy and that "various forms of psychotherapy are equally disappointing" (p. 778). This appears to have been the general perspective on psychotherapy outcome with long-depressed patients suffering from ingrained hopelessness, masochism, and self-sabotage (although such clinical pessimism is rarely stated explicitly). This clinical sentiment is captured in a description of masochistic character by Simons (1987), who distinguishes masochistic character from dysthymic disorder but says the two often overlap:

> They are the patients who unconsciously provoke their therapists either to give up on them, or sadistically abuse them with premature and unempathic interpretations, or pejoratively dismiss them with the misdiagnosis of borderline personality disorder or passive aggressive personality disorder. . . . But whatever the unconscious motives may be in an individual case, the final behavioral outcome is the achievement of what Theodor Reik . . . called "victory through defeat," and often the defeat is a failed psychiatric treatment. (p. 596)

Yet not every clinician believes the prognosis so bleak. We surveyed 43 clinicians and researchers in dysthymia about their experience in treating forms of chronic depression. Thirty-two (74%) responded, including 25 (58%) who completed questionnaires. The latter reported a mean 71% rate of improvement among patients treated either with psychotherapy alone or with a combination of psychotherapy and medication (Markowitz, Moran, & Kocsis, 1990). This impressionistic finding belies the apparently prevailing view of a grim prognosis.

The few existing psychotherapy studies of dysthymic disorder generally suffer from methodological weakness, small sample size, or both. Psychotherapeutic efficacy in these studies should be weighed against the low placebo response rate of dysthymic patients, which is less than 15% (Kocsis, Frances, Voss, Mann, et al., 1988). Methodological variations include the number of psychotherapists involved, the generalizability of their technique, the use of adherence monitoring, and characteristics of the patient population (e.g., inclusion of prior treatment failures). Readers should also note the various definitions of response in these studies and the variation in length of interval before follow-up.

## Psychodynamic Psychotherapy and Psychoanalysis

Recent psychoanalytic literature is meager in its discussion of depression generally and dysthymic disorder in particular (Cohen, Baker, Cohen, Fromm-Reichman, & Weigert, 1954; Jacobson, 1971; Simons, 1987; Stone, 1986). Little effort has been made to differentiate acute and chronic forms of depression. The best psychoanalytic writings (e.g., Arieti & Bemporad, 1978; Bemporad, 1976) have provided rich insights into the minds and feeling states of depressed patients, have suggested interpersonal techniques, but have offered no outcome data. In the 1970s some authors contended that psychodynamic psychotherapy was the treatment of choice for chronic depression (Arieti & Bemporad, 1978; Chodoff, 1972; Jacobson, 1971); unfortunately, there have been no published psychodynamic dysthymia studies, treatment manuals, or trials. Recent reviews of supportive dynamic psychotherapy have not addressed dysthymic disorder (Rockland, 1989, 1993). Hence, although long-term psychodynamic therapy is still frequently prescribed for dysthymic patients, there is no evidence that either short- or long-term psychodynamic treatment benefits such patients. As dysthymia treatment researchers, we hear (from an admittedly select sample of psychodynamic treatment failures) that years of psychodynamic treatment often provide insight about depression but little relief from it.

One potential difficulty with a psychoanalytically oriented approach to dysthymic disorder may involve the confusion of chronic mood state with personality trait. In dysthymic disorder of insidious early onset, whose chronicity has often endured as long as the patient can recall, personality trait and chronic mood disorder have the greatest opportunity to be confused by both patient and therapist. By using a conflictual rather than a medical model of psychopathology, psychoanalytically oriented therapists may tend to blame the victim by assigning the patient responsibility for his or her mood disorder (Cooper, 1985). Dysthymic patients are the first to attribute their problems to a personality defect. Analytic abstinence and neutrality may also be counterproductive for patients whose outlook is so distorted by depressed mood that they may need active support, even therapeutic "cheerleading," to balance their perspective.

## Cognitive-Behavioral Therapy

Cognitive-behavioral therapy (CBT) is a time-limited, structured psychotherapy developed by Beck and colleagues (1979). Its efficacy in treating acute major depression has been demonstrated in multiple clinical trials. The CBT therapist focuses on the "automatic" irrationally negative thoughts that depressed patients report about themselves, their situations, and their future. Through rational discussions with their therapists and written and behavioral homework assignments, patients learn to modify irrationally negative thoughts; as they do, depression decreases.

Several cognitive approaches have been tested in the treatment of dysthymic patients (see Table 9.1). Gonzalez, Lewinsohn, and Clarke (1985) treated 113 patients with 12 individual or group sessions, each 2 hours long, of a skills-training-oriented psychoeducational approach for 2 months, with a follow-up session after 1 month and again at 6 months. More subjects having acute major depression, as defined by Research Diagnostic Criteria (RDC; Spitzer, Endicott, & Robins, 1978), recovered (75%) than did those with (chronic) intermittent depression (43%) or double depression (27%). Recovery was defined as 8 weeks essentially symptom free and a rating of 1 or 2 on the Longitudinal Interval Follow-Up Evaluation (LIFE; Shapiro & Keller, 1979). Follow-up assessments varied between 1 and 3 years. The number of therapists is not stated.

De Jong, Treiber, and Henrich (1986) treated 30 unmedicated inpatients who met DSM-III criteria for both dysthymic disorder and major depression (i.e., double depression) and who had family histories negative for mood disorder. In a 2- to 3-month trial, the combination of activity scheduling, social competence training, and cognitive restructuring yielded a higher response rate (60%) than cognitive restructuring alone (30%) or waiting-list status (10%). Response was defined as meeting two of three criteria: (1)

**TABLE 9.1. Reports of Cognitive-Behavioral Therapy for Dysthymia**

| Study | $n$ | Intensity | Response | Follow-up (months) | Remarks |
|---|---|---|---|---|---|
| Gonzalez, Lewinsohn, & Clarke (1985) | 28 dys.<br>26 double | 12 2-hour sessions in 8 weeks | 43%<br>27% | 12<br>36 | RDC criteria; indiv. or group |
| DeJong, Treiber, & Henrich (1986) | 10 double | 2–3 months inpatient | 60%[a] | 6 | DSM-III criteria; CR and waiting-list comparisons |
| Fennell & Teasdale (1982) | 5 | 20 sessions in 12 weeks | 20% | – | RDC criteria; HRSD 23 → 17 |
| Harpin, Liberman, Marks, Stern, & Bohannon (1982) | 6 | 20 sessions in 10 weeks + 25 mg TCA | 33% | 6 | HRSD 26 → 16; waiting-list control |
| Stravynski, Shahar, & Verreault (1991) | 6 | 15 sessions | 67% | 6 | DSM-III criteria; HRSD 24 → 9 |
| McCullough (1991) | 20 | 14–44 C-BASP sessions | 50% | 24 | DSM-III criteria; 9 remitted at 2 years |
| Mercier, Stewart, & Quitkin (1992) | 8 dys.<br>7 double | 12–16 sessions | 38%<br>43% | 6 | DSM-III criteria |
| Totals | 116 | | 41% | | |

*Note.* $n$ = number of subjects treated; dys., dysthymic; double, double depression; indiv., individual psychotherapy; RDC, Research Diagnostic Criteria; CR, cognitive restructuring; TCA, tricyclic antidepressant; C-BASP, cognitive-behavioral analysis system of psychotherapy.

[a]Three early dropouts omitted from outcome analysis.

a posttreatment Beck Depression Inventory (BDI; Beck, 1978) score of 14 or less, (2) at least a 50% reduction from the pretreatment BDI score, or (3) at least a 50% reduction from the pretreatment score on two relatively obscure treatment scales. Three early dropouts from the two active treatments were omitted from analyses. A 6-month follow-up of a subsample ($n$ = 14) suggested stable treatment effects.

Fennell and Teasdale (1982) treated five subjects who met RDC for major depressive disorder, had a Hamilton Rating Scale for Depression (HRSD; Hamilton, 1960) score of 15 or more ($M$ = 23) and a BDI of 20 or more ($M$ = 31), reported a duration of depression lasting from 18 months—less than the temporal criterion for dysthymic disorder—to 16 years, and had failed to respond to an "adequate trial" (undefined) of antidepressant medication. Therapists with 3½ months of CBT training provided 20 sessions over 4 months. Improvements were described as "modest": The mean HRSD score fell from 22.8 to 17.4, the BDI score fell from 30.8 to 21.4, and only one subject clearly improved (BDI ≤ 9). The authors attributed lack of improvement to "patient characteristics," that is, to the chronicity of their depressive episodes.

Harpin, Liberman, Marks, Stern, and Bohannon (1982) assessed 12 subjects with chronic depression averaging 18 years in duration who had an intake HRSD score of 20 or more and who had failed antidepressant medication. Subjects were alternately assigned to 20 sessions of CBT over 10 weeks or to a waiting-list control. Therapy focused on remediating interpersonal difficulties. Subjects also received 25 mg [*sic*] of tricyclic antidepressant daily. The six subjects receiving active treatment had a significant ($t = 2.37$, $df = 5$, $p < .05$) mean drop in HRSD score from 26.0 ± 6.4 to 16.3 ± 14.6, whereas the mean HRSD score for the waiting-list group did not change. The between-group difference in HRSD change score did not reach statistical significance. At the 6-month follow-up, subjects who had received active treatment still had lowered anxiety ratings, but HRSD scores no longer differed significantly from pretreatment scores. Two of the six treated patients showed major improvement on the HRSD, one of whom maintained this at the 6-month follow-up. No control subjects improved.

Stravynski, Shahar, and Verreault (1991) reported treating six patients with clinically diagnosed DSM-III dysthymic disorder. Therapy consisted of 15 hour-long CBT sessions. Two additional dysthymic subjects diagnosed as having narcissistic and dependent personality disorders were excluded. Independent raters observed significant improvement at termination and at 6-month follow-up: HRSD scores fell from 23.7 ± 2.6 at baseline to 9.3 ± 1.8 posttreatment and to 8.5 ± 9.8 at 6 months. By self-report, BDI scores fell from 26.3 ± 3.1 to 11.7 ± 4.5 posttreatment and to 10.9 ± 8.9 at 6 months. Four subjects no longer met criteria for dysthymic disorder at 15 weeks. The authors inferred that responders had dysthymic disorder with a discrete onset defined by a precipitating life event.

McCullough (1991) described treatment of 10 patients with DSM-III dysthymic disorder using his manualized cognitive-behavioral analysis system of psychotherapy (C-BASP), treatment that entailed a mean 31 ± 9.3 weekly sessions (range 14 to 44). Eight patients met criteria for double depression (J. McCullough, personal communication, April 1993). All reached termination criteria, defined by BDI and Rotter Locus of Control Scale scores of 10 or less. Nine cases remained in remission 2 years later. Of an original cohort of 20 patients, 4 did not complete therapy and the other 6 were unavailable for follow-up; the author did not evaluate their data (J. McCullough, personal communication, May 1993).

Mercier, Stewart, and Quitkin (1992) offered a 12- to 16-week trial of standard CBT to 15 dysthymics (as defined by DSM-III) among a sample of patients with atypical depression. Three of 8 subjects with dysthymic disorder alone and 3 of 7 with double depression responded. All responders had been depressed for at least 7 years. Response to CBT was defined as a Clinical Global Impression (McGlashan, 1973) score of 1 or 2 ("much improved" or "very much improved"), indicating major reduction in psychopathology and no need for additional treatment. For the full cohort of CBT responders, 69% maintained improvement over a 6-month follow-up that included four preplanned booster sessions; the rate of sustained remission among dysthymic patients was not stated.

In summary, seven reports have described cognitive-behavioral treatments of dysthymic disorder. Most treated small idiosyncratic samples (e.g., inpatients, varying degrees of antidepressant nonresponse) and used varying outcome measures. None monitored therapist adherence to the psychotherapy protocol, and most reports (Harpin et al., 1982; McCullough, 1991; Mercier et al., 1992; Stravynski, 1991) reflect the work of a single therapist. Most included some kind of follow-up assessment, an appropriate consideration in the treatment of a chronic disorder. Although results have not been dramatic, they do suggest that some dysthymic patients respond to brief cognitive therapies. In fact, the cumulative response rate of 41% (see Table 9.1) approaches that reported in controlled trials of antidepressant medication (Kocsis, Frances, Voss, Mann, et al., 1988). The paucity of evidence, however, renders hopeful conclusions preliminary.

## *Interpersonal Therapy*

The NIMH Treatment of Depression Collaborative Research Program (Elkin et al., 1989; Sotsky et al., 1991) primarily studied the treatment of major depression but included subjects with double depression (RDC-defined major depression plus chronic minor depression or intermittent depressive disorder). Seventy-one (29.8%) doubly depressed subjects were randomized to treatment with interpersonal therapy (IPT), CBT, imipramine, or placebo; 43 (26.7%) completed the trial. In exploratory analyses, double depression was associated with greater baseline depressive severity and predicted lower placebo response. Double depression was also correlated with higher symptom severity at termination and with incomplete response across treatment conditions. Chronicity and severity of mood disorder thus appeared to predict worse outcome, although not lack of improvement, in standardized treatments for acute major depression.

IPT, like CBT, is a time-limited psychotherapy codified in a manual that has demonstrated efficacy in controlled clinical trials for outpatient major depression and an increasing range of other diagnoses. The patient learns in treatment to recognize links between mood and current interpersonal experiences, focusing on one of four interpersonal problem areas: grief, role dispute, role transition, or interpersonal deficits (Klerman et al., 1984). The therapist explains depression as a medical illness rather than a personality defect, and the patient is given the sick role (Parsons, 1951). IPT has shown benefit in the treatment of acute depression (Elkin et al., 1989; Klerman et al., 1984) as well as in prophylaxis against recurrent major depression (Frank et al., 1990). Interpersonal approaches have been recommended in the treatment of dysthymic disorder (Akiskal, 1990; Cassano, Perugi, Maremmani, & Akiskal, 1990; Goldberg & Bridges, 1990; Hirschfeld, 1990; Weissman & Akiskal, 1984) on the basis of clinical awareness of the interpersonal difficulties dysthymic patients encounter. At Cornell we have developed a manualized approach adapting IPT to dysthymic disorder (IPT-D; Markowitz & Klerman, 1993). Among the adaptations this approach includes is the use of the diagnosis of dysthymic disorder within therapy as a novel form of interpersonal role transition, that is, a role transition that begins with the recognition that one has a chronic mood disorder rather than a melancholy, defective personality. The IPT treatment itself then commences the transition out of chronic depression and into euthymia. Therapists are regularly supervised and monitored for treatment adherence.

Pilot data include three small series of subjects (see Table 9.2). In the first, Mason treated nine dysthymic subjects with IPT: five

**TABLE 9.2. Pilot Treatment Results of Interpersonal Therapy for Dysthymia**

| | | | | | | HRSD scores | | | |
|---|---|---|---|---|---|---|---|---|---|
| Subject | Age | Marital status | Sex | No. of sessions | Sequence | Initial | Final | | Outcome |
| 1 | 46 | Single | F | 16 | S | 19 | 14 | | N |
| 2 | 36 | Div. | F | 16 | S | 24 | 4 | | R |
| 3 | 42 | Div. | F | 3 | S | 24 | 5 | | R |
| 4 | 29 | Div. | F | 11 | S | 16 | 5 | | R |
| 5 | 35 | Single | F | 16 | S | 21 | 13 | | N |
| 6 | 42 | Married | M | 16 | P | 20 | 3 | | R |
| 7 | 36 | Married | M | 5 | P | 27 | 9 | | PR |
| 8 | 38 | Sep. | F | 16 | P | 26 | 9 | | PR |
| 9 | 29 | Single | F | 9 | P | 22 | 3 | | R |
| | | | Seropositive dysthymic subjects | | | | | | |
| 10 | 47 | Cohab. | M | 16 | P | 21 | 4 | | R |
| 11 | 32 | Single | M | 12 | P | 20 | 6 | | R |
| | | | Current cohort | | | | | 6-mo f/u | |
| 12 | 27 | Married | F | 16 | S | 15 | 8 | 2[a] | R |
| 13 | 44 | Married | F | 16 | P | 17 | 4 | 6[b] | R |
| 14 | 26 | Cohab. | F | 16 | P | 22 | 0 | | R |
| 15 | 46 | Married | F | 16 | P | 20 | 8 | | R |
| 16 | 33 | Married | M | 16 | S | 18 | 12 | | N |
| 17 | 40 | Cohab. | M | 16 | P | 33 | 18 | | N |
| Mean | 36.8 | | | 13.5 | | 21.5 | 7.4 | | |
| *SD* | 7.1 | | | 4.3 | | 4.4 | 4.7 | | |

*Note.* Div., divorced; Sep., separated; Cohab., cohabitating; S, IPT subsequent to failed desipramine trial; P, primary IPT without medication; N, nonresponder; R, responder; PR, partial responder; 6-mo f/u, 6-month follow-up.

[a]HRSD = 3 at 8-month follow-up, 5 at 12-month follow-up, 1 at 24-month follow-up.

[b]HRSD = 6 at 8-month follow-up, 6 at 12-month follow-up, 6 at 18-month follow-up.

women who failed to respond to a vigorous desipramine trial and four subjects who refused medication (Mason, Markowitz, & Klerman, 1993). The mean age was 37 (*SD* = 5.4) years. Most of the subjects reported protracted dysthymia (mean duration 22.4 ± 18.9 years, omitting the first 5 years of life). Subjects received 12.0 ± 4.9 sessions of IPT (range 3 to 16). Initial 24-item HRSD scores averaged 19.4 ± 5.0, and scores decreased for all subjects; the mean HRSD score at termination was 7.4 ± 3.8. Compared in quasi-experimental design to randomly chosen dysthymic subjects treated with desipramine, IPT response was equivalent to that of medication.

A separate project that used IPT to treat depressed HIV-seropositive individuals included two dysthymic subjects. These white gay men, ages 47 and 32, reported lifelong depression. Despite the added stress of HIV infection, they improved on HRSD from a mean score of 20.5 at intake to 5.0 at termination of IPT, after 12 and 16 sessions, respectively (Markowitz, Klerman, & Perry, 1992).

We are continuing IPT-D pilot work and testing its replication with additional therapists. Two therapists have thus far completed treatment on six subjects, producing drops in mean HRSD score from 20.8 ± 6.4 (and mean BDI score of 25.2 ± 9.5) at baseline to 8.5 ± 6.3 (with mean BDI score of 12.7 ± 8.2) at termination of acute treatment (Week 16). Responders are generally maintaining their gains when seen in monthly continuation sessions, with follow-up now up to 2 years. Thus, a total of 17 patients, including 7 who had failed vigorous desipramine trials, have received IPT from three therapists. None deteriorated, and 11 (65%) reached remission (HRSD score ≤ 8). Overall, mean HRSD scores fell from 21.5 ± 4.4 at baseline to 7.4 ± 4.7 at acute termination. For IPT, as for CBT, outcome results are limited but encouraging.

## Serial Treatment

The Columbia mood disorders group has raised an interesting question of treatment specificity, namely, whether patients unresponsive to one antidepressant modality may respond to another. Stewart and colleagues (Stewart, Mercier, Agosti, Guardino, & Quitkin, 1993) reported on a subset of CBT nonresponders from the Mercier et al. study who were randomized to treatment with imipramine or placebo. Two pure dysthymics and two double depressives who failed CBT responded to imipramine, whereas two double depressives randomized to placebo did not respond (J. Stewart, personal communication, April 1993).

The sole responder in the Fennell and Teasdale study (1982) and two psychotherapy responders in the study by Harpin and colleagues (1982) had been preselected as medication nonresponders, albeit details of medication trials were not specified and it is possible that they were not truly refractory to medication (Roose & Glassman, 1990). In our studies, seven patients who had not responded to a 10-week trial of high-dosage desipramine improved with IPT. Although these numbers are small indeed, the results imply that medication and psychotherapy may serve complementary purposes in treating differing subtypes of dysthymic patients.

## Combined Treatment

Combined treatment studies are more limited still. Miller and colleagues (Miller, Bishop, Norman, & Keitner, 1985) found that two of four treatment-refractory inpatients with DSM-III double depression responded in an open trial to the combination of either CBT or social skills training (SST) and assorted psychotropic medication (antidepressants or neuroleptics). Patients received a mean 28 psychotherapy sessions over a mean 22 weeks, with sessions provided 5 days per week following an initial 2 weeks of inpatient assessment.

Becker and colleagues (Becker & Heimberg, n.d.; Becker, Heimberg, & Bellack, 1987) reported preliminary results on 39 mildly symptomatic dysthymic subjects randomly assigned in a four-cell study to SST or crisis-supportive psychotherapy and to nortriptyline or placebo. Patients received 16 weekly sessions followed by 2 biweekly sessions. The initial 17-item HRSD mean score was 10.9, declining to 4.5 at termination. Self-report and clinician ratings showed significant improvement for all four treatment conditions.

Waring et al. (1988) described a four-cell randomized treatment trial of 12 mildly depressed women meeting RDC for dysthymia [*sic*] who received 10 weeks of marital cognitive or supportive therapy and doxepin (maximum 150 mg/day) or atropine placebo. All patients improved, with the mean HRSD score falling significantly, from 14.5 to 7.1. Final results have not been reported for either the Becker et al. or the Waring et al. study.

An NIMH Workshop on Combined Medication and Psychotherapy in Depression convened in 1987 in Washington, DC, by Prien and Hirschfeld concluded that discriminating between the antidepressant effects of psychotherapy and pharmacotherapy is difficult because studies indicate that both treatments are effective (i.e., show a "ceiling effect") and because sample sizes in most studies have been small. Patients with chronic depression were deemed an ideal treatment population for differentiating combined and mode-specific treatment effects of antidepressant therapies. The studies have not yet been done.

## Discussion

As yet there have been no large, systematic, controlled clinical trials of the psychotherapy of dysthymic disorder. Data from open trials are promising but scarce. Dysthymic disorder appears increasingly to represent a lingering variant of acute major depression, which has already been shown to respond to antidepressant psychotherapy. As the two mood disorders converge, the argument for testing the efficacy of psychotherapy strengthens. If, as antidepressant medication trials suggest, dysthymic patients are more difficult patients to treat than those with acute major depression, seeking clinical tools to treat them is all the more necessary.

The limited available evidence suggests that, contrary to intuition, brief psychotherapies may effectively treat the chronic mood disorder of dysthymia. In our experience, one advantage of brief therapy is the pressure it puts on both patient and therapist to work actively and quickly while maintaining high treatment expectations. Diagnostic data do corroborate the psychoanalytic perception that masochism is common among dysthymics: We found that 35% of 34 dysthymics met Structured Clinical Interview for DSM-III-R (SCID-II) criteria for self-defeating personality disorder (Markowitz et al., 1992). But do such features indicate a bad prognosis, and do they represent trait or chronic state? It would not be surprising if longer-term therapists, daunted by the grinding chronicity of dysthymic patients, were unwittingly to collude with the dysthymia (Cooper, 1985) by setting lower psychotherapeutic goals, thereby achieving poorer or slower results. High expectations, a medical model of mood disorder, a "here and now" focus on current issues, and the leverage of time-limited therapy may help to jostle patients out of their dysthymic rut. Once relieved of mood disorder, they experience a great release, indeed, a second lease on life.

### Clinical Recommendations

Published evidence supports the use of antidepressant medication as standard treatment for dysthymic disorder. Psychotherapy, whose efficacy data are more limited, may nonetheless offer a reasonable monotherapy, particularly for patients who have not previously received mood-targeted psychotherapy or who refuse medication. If a case of dysthymic disorder does not improve after months of aggressive treatment, however, antidepressant medication should again be considered. A developed therapeutic alliance and the recognition that psychotherapy is not alleviating symptoms may induce a patient who has previously refused medication to try it at this point. Psychotherapy may prove a useful adjunct to medication (Markowitz, 1993).

## Suggestions for Research of Antidysthymic Psychotherapy

### Use of Time-Limited Manualized Psychotherapy

In addition to its therapeutic advantages, brief psychotherapy has clear economic benefits and allows comparison with pharmacological interventions. At least three brief therapies for dysthymic disorder have been delineated in manuals: C-BASP (Stewart et al., 1993), SST (Becker et al., 1987), and IPT (Parsons, 1951). Standard CBT, which has been manualized for treatment of acute depression, appears to have some efficacy for dysthymic disorder as well. The latter three therapies have been used in studies circumscribing time and frequency of sessions.

### Interpersonal Focus

A recurring theme in the studies under review is that psychotherapies tailored for dysthymic disorder seek to address the interpersonal difficulties that are hallmarks of the disorder. This is obviously the focus of IPT, but the description by Harpin et al. (1982) of their cognitive-behavioral approach also stresses an interpersonal approach inasmuch as it provides social skills training in "interpersonal themes," including "refusing unreasonable requests" and "expressing positive feelings to another." Their protocol involved significant others in cases where "the goal of training was to improve the interpersonal interaction and communication between the subject and significant other." SST (Becker et al., 1987) similarly emphasizes interpersonal behavior and social perception. McCullough (1991), while using a different terminology and conceptual approach, also focuses on "$person_1 \times person_2$ interaction" as "the basic subject matter for psychotherapy" (1992, p. 9).

This convergence of treatments reflects the salience of interpersonal difficulties in dysthymic disorder (Hirschfeld, 1990; Kocsis, Frances, Voss, Mason, et al., 1988; Stewart et al., 1988) and the need to address them in antidysthymic psychotherapy. Group or family therapy (Waring et al., 1988) might also help dysthymic patients deal with interpersonal issues.

### Serial Design

Initial controlled treatment trials should assess efficacy of psychotherapy in comparison to a standard reference treatment, that is, antidepressant medication, and to a placebo or other control condition. Because psychotherapy and medication may treat different dysthymic populations, nonresponders to either active treatment might well be crossed over to an open trial of the alternative, as in the study by Stewart et al. (1993).

### Continuation and Maintenance Treatment

Ongoing treatment of psychotherapy responders is warranted, given the chronicity of dysthymic disorder and the risk of relapse and recurrence for mood disorders in general. In this respect psychotherapy and pharmacotherapy of dysthymic disorder probably do not differ. Our limited experience suggests that remitted dysthymic patients greatly appreciate monthly continuation sessions and use the time following acute treatment to consolidate IPT treatment gains. The content of the sessions themselves often appears less relevant than the knowledge that a therapist remains periodically available. The need for ongoing treatment could be tested in a randomized discontinuation trial comparable to the Pittsburgh study of chronic recurrent depression (Frank et al., 1990).

### Combined Treatment Trials

Some may think it premature to compare the combination of psychotherapy and pharmacotherapy to single-modality therapy before the efficacy of psychotherapy for dysthymic patients has been exhaustively proved. Yet even if psychotherapy alone were not to show utility, it might still augment the benefits of antidepressant medication for medication responders (Klerman et al., 1994). "Postdysthymic" medication responders approach but may not attain community levels of social and vocational functioning, at least acutely (Kocsis et al., 1988). They may no longer appear personality disordered (our first two IPT-D responders ceased to meet SCID-II criteria for personality disorder as well as for SCID-P dysthymia; see Chapter 3, this volume), yet they, retarded in their social skills by years of prior depression, may need and benefit from psychotherapy (Markowitz, 1993).

Combined pharmacotherapy and psychotherapy may prove optimal for many dysthymic patients. Psychotherapy has the advantage of empowering patients by giving them the chance to prove to themselves that they can control their mood and their environment. Medication may offer faster relief and surer prophylaxis against recurrence (cf. Frank et al., 1990).

### Follow-Up Assessments

Because dysthymic disorder is by definition chronic, acute treatment outcome may mean less than sustained response on repeated follow-up assessments over 6 months to several years. Follow-up assessment should therefore be included in antidysthymic outcome research.

Psychotherapy research in dysthymic disorder has received relatively little funding. This can be partially explained by the relatively recent development of research psychotherapies, which were initially, and understandably, focused on acute depression. Dysthymic disorder itself has had a doubtful reputation: Although chronic suffering over decades may equal or outweigh the pain of more severe but briefer major depression (Wells et al., 1992), many clinicians and investigators—and perhaps the patients themselves—seem to view dysthymic disorder with suspicion, that is, 23 to consider it a "soft" diagnosis. The diagnostic system is biased by a tyranny of the acute inasmuch as it defines "major" depression by severity of current symptoms and relegates severity of duration to the "subsyndromal," and, by analogy, "minor." Yet, paradoxically, chronicity of symptoms may daunt psychotherapists who treat dysthymic disorder.

The distinction between pure dysthymic disorder and double depression may have received more attention than it deserves. Some studies (e.g., Becker & Heimberg, n.d.) have foundered in the pursuit of "pure" dysthymic patients. Yet the DSM-IV field trials found that 79% of dysthymic patients eventually develop the couple of additional symptom criteria they need for a diagnosis of major depression, thus qualifying for the label of double depression (McCullough, Klein, Shea, & Miller, 1992). What may be largely an artifactual difference in severity criteria (Kocsis & Frances, 1987) may hold less prognostic and diagnostic importance than the chronicity of the mood disorder. The pure dysthymic disorder double depression distinction should not be a barrier to research, although researchers should control for double depression in their statistical analyses.

Both growing awareness of the public health significance of dysthymic disorder and the availability of treatment technology make the time ripe to answer Weissman and Akiskal's (1984) proposal for antidysthymic psychotherapy trials.

## Summary

Psychotherapy of dysthymic disorder has received too little serious attention and funding. Impressive advances in the pharmacotherapy of dysthymic disorder should not obscure the need for psychosocial treatments for the 50% of patients who do not respond to medication. Despite the dearth of psychotherapy outcome studies in this area, extant data do suggest that relatively brief focal antidepressant psychotherapies may successfully treat many patients with lifelong mood disorders. Research should involve manualized, time-limited therapies with an interpersonal focus and should consider serial designs as well as maintenance therapy to ensure the persistence of treatment gains. Psychotherapy may also be a helpful adjunct to antidepressant medication.

### Acknowledgments

This chapter was presented in part at the NIMH Workshop on Subsyndromal Mood Disorders: Dysthymia and Cyclothymia, Bethesda, MD, April 1993; at the 146th annual meeting of the American Psychiatric

Association, San Francisco, May 1993; and at the NIMH Workshop on the Effectiveness and Cost of Psychotherapy, McLean, VA, January 1994.

It is adapted from Markowitz (1994). Copyright 1994 by the American Psychiatric Association. Adapted by permission.

Preparation of this chapter was supported in part by Grant No. MH-19069 from the National Institute of Mental Health.

## References

Akiskal, H. S. (1981). Subaffective disorders: Dysthymic, cyclothymic and bipolar II disorders in the "borderline" realm. *Psychiatric Clinics of North America*, *4*, 25–46.

Akiskal, H. S. (1990). Towards a definition of dysthymia: Boundaries with personality and mood disorders. In S. W. Burton & H. S. Akiskal (Eds.), *Dysthymic disorder* (pp. 1–12). London: Gaskell.

Akiskal, H. S., Rosenthal, T. L., Haykal, R. F., Lemmi, H., Rosenthal, R. H., & Scott-Strauss, A. (1980). Characterological depressions: Clinical and sleep EEG findings separating "subaffective dysthymias" from "character spectrum disorders." *Archives of General Psychiatry*, *37*, 777–783.

American Psychiatric Association. (1980). *Diagnostic and statistical manual of mental disorders*. Washington, DC: Author.

American Psychiatric Association. (1987). *Diagnostic and statistical manual of mental disorders* (3rd ed., rev.). Washington, DC: Author.

American Psychiatric Association. (1994). *Diagnostic and statistical manual of mental disorders* (4th ed.). Washington, DC: Author.

Arieti, S., & Bemporad, J. (1978). *Severe and mild depressions*. New York: Basic Books.

Beck, A. T. (1978). *Depression Inventory*. Philadelphia: Center for Cognitive Therapy.

Beck, A. T., Rush, A. J., Shaw, B. F., & Emery, G. (1979). *Cognitive therapy of depression*. New York: Guilford Press.

Becker, R. E., & Heimberg, R. G. (n.d.). *Dysthymia: Preliminary results of treatment with social skills training, crisis supportive psychotherapy, nortriptyline, and placebo*. Unpublished manuscript, Medical College of Pennsylvania.

Becker, R. E., Heimberg, R. G., & Bellack, A. S. (1987). *Social skills training treatment for depression*. New York: Pergamon.

Bemporad, J. (1976). Psychotherapy of the depressive character. *Journal of the American Academy of Psychoanalysis*, *4*, 347–372.

Cassano, G. B., Perugi, G., Maremmani, I., & Akiskal, H. S. (1990). Social adjustment in dysthymia. In S. W. Burton & H. S. Akiskal (Eds.), *Dysthymic disorder* (pp. 78–85). London: Gaskell.

Chodoff, P. (1972). The depressive personality: A critical review. *Archives of General Psychiatry, 25*, 666–673.

Cohen, M. B., Baker, G., Cohen, R. A., Fromm-Reichman, F., & Weigert, E. V. (1954). An intensive study of twelve cases of manic–depressive psychosis. *Psychiatry, 17*, 103–137.

Cooper, A. M. (1985). Will neurobiology influence psychoanalysis? *American Journal of Psychiatry, 142*, 1395–1402.

de Jong, R., Treiber, R., & Henrich, G. (1986). Effectiveness of two psychological treatments for inpatients with severe and chronic depressions. *Cognitive Therapy and Research, 10*, 645–663.

Elkin, I., Shea, M. T., Watkins, J. T., Imber, S. D., Sotsky, S. M., Collins, J. F., Glass, D. R., Pilkonis, P. A., Leber, W. R., Docherty, J. P., Fiester, S. J., & Parloff, M. B. (1989). National Institute of Mental Health Treatment of Depression Collaborative Research Program: General effectiveness of treatments. *Archives of General Psychiatry, 46*, 971–982.

Fennell, M. J. V., & Teasdale, J. D. (1982). Cognitive therapy with chronic, drug-refractory depressed outpatients. A note of caution. *Cognitive Therapy and Research, 6*, 455–460.

Frank, E., Kupfer, D. J., Perel, J. M., Cornes, C., Jarrett, D. B., Mallinger, A. G., Thase, M. E., McEachran, A. B., & Grochocinski, V. J. (1990). Three-year outcomes for maintenance therapies in recurrent depression. *Archives of General Psychiatry, 47*, 1093–1099.

Goldberg, D. P., & Bridges, K. W. (1990). Epidemiological observations on the concept of dysthymic disorder. In S. W. Burton & H. S. Akiskal (Eds.), *Dysthymic disorder* (pp. 104–111). London: Gaskell.

Gonzalez, L. R., Lewinsohn, P. M., & Clarke, G. N. (1985). Longitudinal follow-up of unipolar depressives: An investigation of predictors of relapse. *Journal of Consulting and Clinical Psychology*, 53, 461–469.

Hamilton, M. (1960). A rating scale for depression. *Journal of Neurology, Neurosurgery, and Psychiatry, 25*, 56–62.

Harpin, R. E., Liberman, R. P., Marks, I., Stern, S., & Bohannon, W. E. (1982). Cognitive-behavior therapy for chronically depressed patients: A controlled pilot study. *Journal of Nervous and Mental Disease, 170*, 295–301.

Harrison, W. M., & Stewart, J. W. (1993). Pharmacotherapy of dysthymia. *Psychiatric Annals, 23*, 638–648.

Hirschfeld, R. M. A. (1990). Personality and dysthymia. In S. W. Burton & H. S. Akiskal (Eds.), *Dysthymic disorder* (pp. 69–77). London: Gaskell.

Howland, R. H. (1991). Pharmacotherapy of dysthymia. *Journal of Clinical Psychopharmacology, 11*, 83–92.

Jacobson, E. (1971). *Depression.* New York: International Universities Press.

Keller, M. B., Lavori, P. W., Endicott, J., Coryell, W., & Klerman, G. L (1983). "Double depression": Two-year follow-up. *American Journal of Psychiatry, 140*, 689–694.

Kessler, R. C., McGonagle, K. A., Zhao, S., Nelson, C. B., Hughes, M., Eshleman, S., Wittchen, H.-U., & Kendler, K. S. (1994). Lifetime and 12-month prevalence of DSM-III-R psychiatric disorders in the United States: Results from the National Comorbidity Study. *Archives of General Psychiatry, 51*, 8–19.

Klerman, G. L., Weissman, M. M., Markowitz, J., Glick, I., Wilner, P. J., Mason, B., & Shear, M. K. (1994). Medication and psychotherapy. In A. E. Bergin & S. L. Garfield (Eds.), *Handbook of psychotherapy and behavior change* (4th ed., pp. 734–782). New York: Wiley.

Klerman, G. L., Weissman, M. M., Rounsaville, B. J., & Chevron, E. S. (1984). *Interpersonal psychotherapy of depression.* New York: Basic Books.

Kocsis, J. H., & Frances, A. J. (1987). A critical discussion of DSM-III dysthymic disorder. *American Journal of Psychiatry, 144*, 1534–1542.

Kocsis, J. H., Frances, A. J., Voss, C., Mann, J. J., Mason, B. J., & Sweeney, J. (1988). Imipramine treatment for chronic depression. *Archives of General Psychiatry, 45*, 253–257.

Kocsis, J. H., Frances, A. J., Voss, C., Mason, B. J., Mann, J. J., & Sweeney, J. (1988). Imipramine and social-vocational adjustment in chronic depression. *American Journal of Psychiatry, 145*, 997–999.

Markowitz, J. C. (1993). Psychotherapy of the post-dysthymic patient. *Journal of Psychotherapy Practice and Research, 2*, 157–163.

Markowitz, J. C. (1994). Psychotherapy of dysthymia. *American Journal of Psychiatry, 151*, 1114–1121.

Markowitz, J. C., & Klerman, G. L. (1993). *Manual for interpersonal therapy of dysthymia* (version 2.1). New York: Cornell University Medical College, Department of Psychiatry.

Markowitz, J. C., Klerman, G. L., & Perry, S. (1992). Interpersonal psychotherapy of depressed HIV-seropositive outpatients. *Hospital and Community Psychiatry, 43*, 885–890.

Markowitz, J. C., Moran, M. E., & Kocsis, J. H. (1990, May). *Does psychotherapy treat chronic depression?* Paper presented at the 146th annual meeting of the American Psychiatric Association, New York.

Markowitz, J. C., Moran, M. E., Kocsis, J. H., & Frances, A. J. (1992). Prevalence and comorbidity of dysthymic disorder among psychiatric outpatients. *Journal of Affective Disorders, 24*, 63–71.

Mason, B. J., Markowitz, J. C., & Klerman, G. L. (1993). IPT for dysthymic disorder. In G. L. Klerman & M. M. Weissman (Eds.), *New applications of interpersonal therapy* (pp. 225–264). Washington, DC: American Psychiatric Press.

McCullough, J. P. (1991). Psychotherapy for dysthymia: A naturalistic study of ten patients. *Journal of Nervous and Mental Disease, 179,* 734–740.

McCullough, J. P. (1992). *The manual for therapists treating the chronic depressions and using the cognitive-behavioral analysis system of psychotherapy.* Unpublished manuscript, Virginia Commonwealth University, Department of Psychology.

McCullough, J. P., Klein, D. N., Shea, M. T., & Miller, I. (1992, September). *Review of DSM-IV mood disorder data in the field trials.* Paper presented at the 100th meeting of the American Psychological Association, Washington, DC.

McGlashan, T. (Ed.). (1973). *The documentation of Clinical Psychotropic Drug Trial.* Rockville, MD: National Institute of Mental Health.

Mercier, M. A., Stewart, J. W., & Quitkin, F. M. (1992). A pilot sequential study of cognitive therapy and pharmacotherapy of atypical depression. *Journal of Clinical Psychiatry, 53,* 166–170.

Miller, I. W., Bishop, S. B., Norman, W. H., & Keitner, G. I. (1985). Cognitive/behavioural therapy and pharmacotherapy with chronic, drug-refractory depressed inpatients: A note of optimism. *Behavioural Psychotherapy, 13,* 320–327.

Parsons, T. (1951). Illness and the role of the physician: A sociological perspective. *American Journal of Orthopsychiatry, 21,* 452–460.

Rockland, L. H. (1989). *Supportive therapy.* New York: Basic Books.

Rockland, L. H. (1993). A review of supportive psychotherapy, 1986–1992. *Hospital and Community Psychiatry, 44,* 1053–1060.

Roose, S. P., & Glassman, A. H. (Eds.). (1990). *Treatment strategies for refractory depression.* Washington, DC: American Psychiatric Press.

Shapiro, R., & Keller, M. (1979). *Longitudinal Interval Follow-Up Evaluation (LIFE).* Unpublished manuscript, Massachusetts General Hospital.

Simons, R. C. (1987). Psychoanalytic contributions to psychiatric nosology: Forms of masochistic behavior. *Journal of the American Psychoanalytic Association,* 35, 583–608.

Sotsky, S. M., Glass, D. R., Shea, M. T., Pilkonis, P. A., Collins, J. F., Elkin, I., Watkins, J. T., Imber, S. D., Leber, W. R., Moyer, J., & Oliveri, M. E. (1991). Patient predictors of response to psychotherapy and pharmacothernpy: Findings in the NIMH Treatment of Depression Collaborative Research Program. *American Journal of Psychiatry, 148,* 997–1008.

Spitzer, R. L., Endicott, J., & Robins, E. (1978). *Research Diagnostic Criteria (RDC) for a selected group of functional disorders* (3rd ed.). New York: New York State Psychiatric Institute, Biometrics Research.

Stewart, J. W., Mercier, M. A., Agosti, V., Guardino, M., & Quitkin, F. M. (1993). Imipramine is effective after unsuccessful cognitive therapy: Sequential use of cognitive therapy and imipramine in depressed outpatients. *Journal of Clinical Psychopharmacology, 13*, 114–119.

Stewart, J. W., Quitkin, F. M., McGrath, P. J., Rabkin, J. G., Markowitz, J. S., Tricamo, E., & Klein, D. F. (1988). Social functioning in chronic depression: Effect of 6 weeks of antidepressant treatment. *Psychiatry Research, 25*, 213–222.

Stone, L. (1986). Psychoanalytic observations on the pathology of depressive illness: Selected spheres of ambiguity or disagreement. *Journal of the American Psychoanalytic Association, 34*, 329–362.

Stravynski, A., Shahar, A., & Verreault, R. (1991). A pilot study of the cognitive treatment of dysthymic disorder. *Behavioural Psychotherapy, 4*, 369–372.

Waring, E. M., Chamberlaine, C. H., McCrank, E. W., Stalker, C. A., Carver, C., Fry, R., & Barnes, S. (1988). Dysthymia: A randomized study of cognitive marital therapy and antidepressants. *Canadian Journal of Psychiatry, 33*, 96–99.

Weissman, M. M., & Akiskal, H. S. (1984). The role of psychotherapy in chronic depressions: A proposal. *Comprehensive Psychiatry, 25*, 23–31.

Weissman, M. M., Leaf, P. J., Bruce, M. L., & Florio, L. (1988). The epidemiology of dysthymia in five communities: Rates, risks, comorbidity, and treatment. *American Journal of Psychiatry, 145*, 815–819.

Wells, K. B., Burnam, M. A., Rogers, W., Hays, R., & Camp, P. (1992). The course of depression in adult outpatients: Results from the Medical Outcomes Study. *Archives of General Psychiatry, 49*, 788–794.

Wells, K. B., Stewart, A., Hays, R. D., Burnam, A., Rogers, W., Daniels, M., Berry, S., Greenfield, S., & Ware, J. (1989). The functioning and well-being of depressed patients: Results from the Medical Outcomes Study. *Journal of the American Medical Association, 262*, 914–919.

# *Editors' Afterword*

JAMES H. KOCSIS
DANIEL N. KLEIN

The recent development of a wide range of safe and effective antidepressant medications has encouraged a shift in focus in the treatment of milder forms of depression in outpatient settings. This shift has captured a great deal of attention in the popular media and has spawned a best-selling book, *Listening to Prozac* (Kramer, 1993), by a clinical psychiatrist in private practice. Nosological considerations relevant to clinical decisions about treatment of depression have also changed. In an earlier era of psychiatric therapeutics, clinicians attended to issues of symptom severity and to cross-sectional symptom profiles that attempted to differentiate psychotic, endogenous, and atypical subtypes of depression. The important decisions concerned hospitalization, the use of electroconvulsive therapy, and the choice between tricyclic antidepressants and monoamine oxidase inhibitors.

Several factors have converged to change the decision-making algorithms used in the treatment of depression. These have included more attention to the course and natural history of the illness and the demonstration that chronic forms of depression–whether mild (i.e., pure dysthymic disorder) or severe (i.e., double depression)–can benefit remarkably from adequate medication. It has been demonstrated that the benefit of pharmacotherapy extends beyond the reduction of depressive symptoms. Social and interpersonal function and even personality traits appear to improve in many instances. Patients who have been chronically avoidant, socially phobic, or self-defeating may improve social performance, increase assertive behavior, and achieve important changes in their performance at work and in their interpersonal relations. The relative safety and minimal side effects of some of the newer drugs make them relatively simple to prescribe, which leads to clinical and philosophical questions about the definition of "caseness" and the threshold for prescribing medication. The newer drugs, however, are not a panacea. Some chronically depressed patients do not respond to treatment with medication. Surprisingly, little has been found to predict response. It is not known whether prior psychotherapy is a factor in drug response, nor do we know the value of concurrent psychotherapy in enhancement or facilitation of pharmacotherapy. Finally, these newer drugs may have side effects (e.g., sexual dysfunction is associated with serotonin reuptake inhibitors), which are less tolerable when longer-term treatment is required. The indicated duration of treatment and the effects of discontinuation of treatment are other important areas of current and future research in the treatment of chronic depression.

Noteworthy accomplishments have been made in the epidemiology of dysthymic disorder in both community and clinical settings, in the delineation of comorbid psychiatric diagnoses, and in understanding the associated social and interpersonal impairments. The methodology for research in chronic depression has been advanced by development of more reliable and valid diagnostic criteria and by the development of assessment techniques specifically designed for this population.

Nonetheless, despite all of the work summarized in the excellent reviews by our authors, there are still numerous gaps in our knowledge. Much work remains to be done. By necessity and by design, initial efforts to investigate the epidemiology, course, and comorbidity of dysthymic disorder have utilized cross-sectional assessments of retrospective history. Such studies have indicated that the dysthymic syndrome usually begins in childhood or adolescence and may become complicated by superimposed major depressive episodes, personality disorders, substance abuse, or other psychiatric diagnoses. Kovacs and colleagues (Kovacs, Feinberg, Crouse-Novak, & Finkelstein, 1984) have pioneered in the development of a prospective longitudinal approach to studies of depressive disorders in childhood. This type of study promises to shed much more light on the natural history, course, and comorbidity of dysthymic disorder in the future.

There have also been preliminary indications from studies of family history (Akiskal, King, Rosenthal, Robinson, & Scott-Strauss, 1981; Klein, Taylor, Dickstein, & Harding, 1988) that dysthymic disorder may be associated with a high familial prevalence of unipolar (and possibly bipolar) affective illness. Methodologically rigorous family studies conducted with dysthymic probands and appropriate comparison groups are currently under way. If the familial linkage of dysthymic disorder and recurrent major depression is supported, future genetic research in affective disorders may be warranted. Similarly, if dysthymic disorder proves to be the clinical "trait" of recurrent major affective illness, studies of biological trait markers should be undertaken in dysthymic cases at various phases of the disorder.

Finally, from the standpoint of research on the treatment of dysthymic disorder, most progress has occurred in studies of short-term pharmacotherapy. It appears that all of the major classes of antidepressant medication hold promise for the treatment of this illness. Furthermore, dysthymic disorder has responded relatively poorly to placebo in controlled clinical trials. Studies of long-term treatment are important and are currently in progress.

A most intriguing and important issue is the as-yet-undefined role of psychotherapy in the treatment of dysthymic disorder. Studies are needed to examine the effectiveness of various forms of short- and long-term psychotherapy both alone and in combination with pharmacotherapy.

## References

Akiskal, H. S., King, D., Rosenthal, T. L., Robinson, D., & Scott-Strauss, A. (1981). Chronic depressions: Clinical and familial characteristics in 137 probands. *Journal of Affective Disorders, 3*, 297–315.

Klein, D. N., Taylor, E. B., Dickstein, S. & Harding, K. (1988). Primary, early-onset dysthymia: Comparison with primary nonbipolar nonchronic major depression on demographic, clinical, familial, personality, and socioenvironmental characteristics and short-term outcome. *Journal of Abnormal Psychology, 97*, 387–398.

Kovacs, M., Feinberg, T. L., Crouse-Novak, M. A., & Finkelstein, R. (1984). Depressive disorders in childhood: I. A longitudinal prospective study of characteristics and recovery. *Archives of General Psychiatry, 41*, 229–237.

Kramer, P. D. (1993). *Listening to Prozac.* New York: Viking Press.

# Index